THE
LITTLE
LOCKSMITH

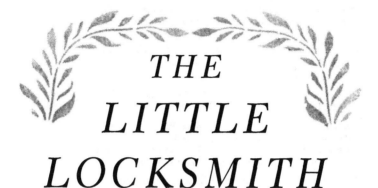

THE
LITTLE
LOCKSMITH

A MEMOIR

BY

KATHARINE BUTLER HATHAWAY

Foreword by Alix Kates Shulman
Afterword by Nancy Mairs

Un labeur courageux muni d'humble constance
Resiste à tous assauts par douce pacience

PLANTIN

THE FEMINIST PRESS
AT THE CITY UNIVERSITY OF NEW YORK

Published by The Feminist Press at The City University of New York
The Graduate Center, 365 Fifth Avenue, New York, NY 10016, feministpress.org
First Feminist Press edition, 2000

Library of Congress Cataloging-in-Publication Data
Hathaway, Katharine Butler, 1890–1942

 The little locksmith : a memoir / Katharine Butler Hathaway ; foreword by Alix Kates
Shulman ; afterword by Nancy Mairs

  p. cm.

 Originally published: New York : Coward-McCann, 1942.

 ISBN 1-55861-238-6 (cloth : alk. paper) — ISBN 1-55861-239-4 (paper : alk. paper)

  1. Hathaway, Katharine Butler, 1890–1942. 2. Authors, American—20th century—Biography. 3. Pott's disease—Patients—Biography. 4. Women—Maine—Castine—
Biography. 5. Castine (Me.)—Biography. I. Title.

PS3515.A8615 Z465 2000
362.4'3'092—dc21
[B]   00-020345

The Feminist Press is grateful to Helene D. Goldfarb, Joanne Markell, Genevieve Vaughan,
and Patricia L. Wentworth and Mark Fagan for their generosity in supporting this publication.

Design for the original edition by Carl Purlington Rollins, set in Caledonia type, with deco-
rations adapted from old stencils
Front and back matter typeset by Dayna Navaro, using stencils from the original edition
Printed on acid-free paper by Transcontinental Printing
Printed in Canada

08 07 06 05 04 03   5 4 3

CONTENTS

FOREWORD

In the early 1980s, soon after I had moved alone to the coast of Maine where my life unexpectedly expanded and deepened, my daughter gave me a copy of *The Little Locksmith*. Behind the misleading title (this is definitely not a children's book), among the discards in the forty-eight-cent bin of New York City's largest secondhand bookstore, she had discerned a rare treasure and, after reading it, inscribed it to me for my birthday. The story of a woman who, in defiance of all expectations for someone of her circumstances and gender, buys a house on the Maine coast and transforms a life of doom into one of triumph was a perfect gift to me.

Holding its own among the best spiritual autobiographies of our time, this "story of the liberation of a human being," as its author describes it, so moved me that I wanted to shower copies of it on my friends, promote its republication, teach it to my students, and find out all I could about its author, her life and work. Fortunately, secondhand copies were easy to come by since the book had been a bestseller in 1943 and a main selection of the Book-of-the-Month Club and had even been excerpted in the *Atlantic Monthly* before publication, during the dark days of World War II. But like so many valuable literary works by women, not many years after the author's death (at age fifty-two, on the very eve of the publication of her memoir), the book languished in attics and was forgotten. I began to buy up enough copies to supply my classes, bless my friends, and quell my fear of running out. But sometimes I found myself down to my last copy and had to begin collecting again. It is therefore with relief, as well as enthusiasm, that I now, these many years after my first memorable encounter with *The Little Locksmith*, relish the opportunity to introduce to a whole new spectrum of readers Katharine Butler Hathaway's masterwork. And how fitting that The Feminist Press, an institution that has faithfully returned to print so many important forgotten books by women, is its new publisher.

Born in 1890 into a loving, well-to-do Massachusetts family, Katharine Butler came of age as a member of that bold generation of educated, somewhat bohemian modern women who were the first to bob their hair, openly embrace sex, question marriage, revere art, and claim a right to every sort of experience and accomplishment. But because Katharine's tubercular spine did not grow normally (though the "terrible"—and, to her, unspeakable—word *hunchback* was not among such self-descriptions as "deformed," "invalid," "belonging to the company of the queer, the maimed, the unfit," and, most delicately, "a very small childish spinster") it was not expected that she would participate in the vital social and sexual passions of her times. When the teenaged Katharine, having spent the central decade of her childhood bedridden and strapped to a stretcher, realized the limitations that would be imposed upon her life, she was stricken with despair.

Not that she lacked the spirit, talent, or discipline to achieve her burgeoning ambition of asserting herself through writing. (And among the many charms of this book are passages of uncommon wisdom about the writing vocation: the need for patience, humility, solitude, and devotion. Not for nothing did she choose Flaubert as her master.) But the grotesque disparity between her own "sparkling," expansive sense of herself in solitude and the "painful narrow . . . identity that had been created for me by others"—views that she knew "could not exist inside the same body at the same time"—presented an excruciating challenge. To meet that challenge, to "outwit fate" by asserting her own self-created vision in the face of the world's cruel dismissal and her own shame and fear and anguish, became the central drama of her life, which is recounted in this powerful and inspiring work.

This is also a book about a house—a surprisingly large one for "a very small childish spinster"—overlooking Penobscot Bay in Castine, Maine. There, in her thirties, after a lifetime of being hovered over and protected like a child, Hathaway took control of her own destiny by using a legacy to purchase a house where, she exults, she could at last be "alone and free." Having acquired her house without advice or help from family or friends—indeed against all their expectations—she determined "to find out what I really was" and "begin to live." In an era when it was still an act of defiance for a woman—even a woman mature enough to be labeled "spinster"—to choose to live alone according to her own unconventional lights, Hathaway's adventure was dense with symbolic meaning, so much so that twice I made the pilgrimage to Castine to experience firsthand the site of her extraordinary spiritual triumph and literary mastery.

The very style she perfected there, somehow spare and extravagant at once, exudes her expanding sense of accomplishment. Eschewing the frivolous or trifling in order to distill the pure emotional essence of her experience, she renders into words both subtleties and extremes of feeling seldom encountered outside the bravest spiritual autobiographies. Each event she recounts is full of consequence. This strategy keeps the intensity of her narrative mounting page by page. Seven years in the writing (1935–42), this riveting account of the transformation of a life ends with an epilogue in which Hathaway forthrightly confesses, "I love this book and can hardly bear to leave it." Rereading it yet again, I know just what she means.

There is in fact much more to know of Katharine Butler Hathaway after the events of the final chapter of this book (for which she planned two sequels): the long denied sexual fulfillment, a stint in expatriate Paris among the avant-garde artists and bohemians she considered her true peers, romance and marriage, and finally the literary recognition she craved. But although another volume of her writing does exist—a posthumously edited miscellany of journal entries, poems, letters, and drawings—there is no sequel to *The Little Locksmith*.

No matter. This single profound work is treasure enough.

Alix Kates Shulman
Long Island, Maine
September 1999

THE
LITTLE
LOCKSMITH

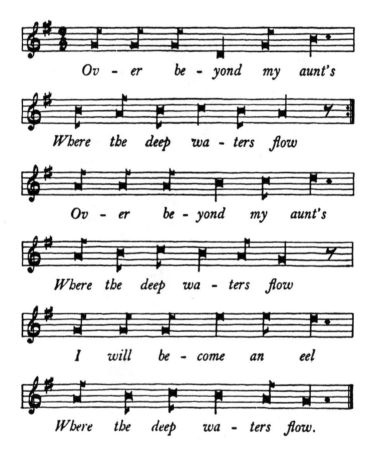

Ov - er be - yond my aunt's

Where the deep wa - ters flow

Ov - er be - yond my aunt's

Where the deep wa - ters flow

I will be - come an eel

Where the deep wa - ters flow.

A SONG OF
TRANSFORMATIONS

Over beyond my aunt's
Where the deep waters flow
I will become an eel
Where the deep waters flow.

If you become an eel
Where the deep waters flow
Angler I then shall turn
That I may get you so.

Angler if you should turn
That you may get me so
I will become a lark
Over the fields to go.

If you become a lark
Over the fields to go
Hunter I then shall turn
That I may get you so.

Hunter if you should turn
That you may get me so
I will become your bride
For that you love me so.

THE LITTLE LOCKSMITH

1

I HAVE an island in the palm of my right hand. It is quite large and shaped like an almond. To make this island, the fate line splits in two in the middle, then comes together again up toward the Mount of Jupiter. I don't know what an island means in palmistry. No two people ever interpret it alike. But it looks to me, and that is enough for me, as if it meant that a quiet respectable fate were suddenly going to explode in the middle of life into something entirely new and strange, and then be folded together again and go on as quietly as it began. And because something of this kind has happened to me I get a rather foolish magic-loving satisfaction from believing that my island represents that period, the cycle of precious experience which befell me and which I am going to write about in this book. I treasure that little thing in my hand. I pore over it reminiscently, gratefully. I like to know it is there. It is the lucky coin that saved me. It is the wafer of beneficent magic that made everything all right at last. It is the yeast that made my life rise.

1

The Little Locksmith

When I was young I was so sure of the marvelous way my life was going to unfold that I never wasted my time looking for signs and portents. But something went wrong. The future I expected didn't come, and so I began to be superstitious and sometimes took a furtive look at the palm of my hand when I was alone. And there I found the curious and possibly hopeful island. If the subject of fortune-telling came up in a roomful of people I secretly hungered for my turn. I put on a cool, superior air as I watched the others, and I made an exaggerated pretense of being reluctant and skeptical when my turn came—while inwardly of course I was no more reluctant and skeptical than any other ambitious willful people are in the late twenties, and then in the early thirties, and then in the middle thirties, if their lives are being held at a complete standstill during those heartbreakingly precious years. As foolishly and fiercely as I had believed in myself, so foolishly and fiercely I came to believe in gypsies, astrologers, card-readers, crystal-gazers, or anyone else who would give me any hope. And as each year dropped off my life I felt an almost unbearable longing to know what the great thing could be that was going to happen to me when I reached that amazing island in the palm of my hand.

Now I know what it was. It has happened. And it really was an island. The things that happened there made a period that was complete in itself, and so separate from the rest of my life that it was almost unrecognizable as mine. It was a period that seemed unreal and half enchanted, because it was so foreign to me and to everything that I had thought and been before. It floated like an island in the rest of my life.

2

The Little Locksmith

Since then I have been thinking about islands, those explosions of apparently uncharacteristic experience that occur in certain lives. Most of the people we know are terribly afraid of such islands. They see one looming ahead and they hurriedly steer off in another direction. In order to save one's life, as has been said, one must be willing to let it be tossed away, and not many of us are willing. All well-brought-up people are afraid of having any experience which seems to them uncharacteristic of themselves as they imagine themselves to be. Yet this is the only kind of experience that is really alive and can lead them anywhere worth going. New, strange, uncharacteristic, uncharted experience, coming at the needed moment, is sometimes as necessary in a person's life as a plough in a field. Yet those people who are most capable of continuous development, because of their rich and fastidious and subtle natures, seem to feel a passionate fear and resentment of any really new experience. Change must always come, to them and in them, evenly and slowly and always in a given direction. If it takes a sudden sharp turn, or seems to be leading them into a place that they think is not fit for them, they refuse to follow it. Oh, lucky beyond most human beings is the refined and well-brought-up person who comes upon an utterly unfamiliar island flat in the middle of his fate line, and who is bold and crazy enough to defy the almost overwhelming chorus of complacency and inertia and other people's ideas and to follow the single, fresh, living voice of his own destiny, which at the crucial moment speaks aloud to him and tells him to come on.

3

Then what happens is like the Japanese fairy tale of the man who visited a lady in her palace under the sea. It is romance, and it becomes legend. One reaches the island, is tossed ashore and stays one's allotted time, and one leaves the island in the end. One leaves it, but the island floats there still, separate from all the rest of one's life, foreign and almost incredible. But there it is, and it is enough that it is there, even though one can never go back to it again. As one looks back upon it, it comes to seem like an allegorical tale. It throws light on everything that went before, and on everything that comes afterward. One recognizes it as the true heart of one's life, for without it one's life would have been empty. Some fortunate lives unfold without obstruction or flaw, and these do not need islands.

2

I WAS coming very close to my own island when I reached the quiet refined age of just past thirty. And by that time I had lost all interest in the little mark in my hand as a promise of adventure or change for me. By that time change was the thing I wanted least of all. I had suffered an unbearable thirst and hunger for experience, and I had been caught and held by my predicament in such a way that I could not seek what I needed and it could not come to me. Therefore at last I turned my back on myself and my predicament in the hope of turning my back on any more unbearable disappointment and despair.

I decided that I would be a writer, and I determined to be the kind of writer, like Flaubert, who removes everything from his life except his writing in order that his writing may live and he may live in it. I even killed in myself any desire that writing should bring me success or fame. I would never risk again any sort of disappointment. Personal obscurity and infinite patience and infinite devotion were to be my program. I knew very well that out of these I could build and maintain a delight as intense as the mystic delight of any nun who has renounced the world.

And so I combined an absolutely uneventful outward personal life with a vivid life of imaginary experience. I filled notebook after notebook with ideas for stories and things in Nature I had noticed and adored, and all kinds of things, minute and spectacular, that I saw happening in other people's lives. As they grew, my notebooks became as secretly precious to me as their slowly growing honeycomb must be to a hive of bees. And I adored, idolized even, the piece of work which was always in progress—the one whole imaginary experience in the form of a novel or a long short story, which was always in the process of unfolding before the intensely fascinated gaze of my mind's eye. This mysteriously organic growing thing held the essence of life for me, as I concentrated upon it all the skill I had and all my love. I clung to it the way a bee clings to a flower, clutching at it with my whole body and mind, absorbing it and being absorbed by it as though I would die if I let go. And it seemed as if I would die, if I lost it or lost my power to cling to it. When I was separated from it for a few days, or sometimes even for a single day, my life became an abyss which terrified me, an unfamiliar place where I had a sense of never being at home, of never really belonging there. Because of this queer unnatural suffering, I feared and dreaded any external change which might threaten to prevent me from clinging tight to my great anesthetizing flower of dreams. And when I began to entertain at first mildly and then eagerly the innocent idea that it would be very nice to have a house of my own it was mainly for the sake, I thought, of making this secret life of mine safer still from external interference. I was intending to make it very hard indeed for anything to dislodge or disturb me.

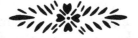

3

SO I began to peer among lilac bushes and old apple trees as I went along country roads looking for my house. I thought I knew the sort of house I wanted and that would be suitable for me. It would be dark and weather-beaten on the outside and have small curved windowpanes and a mossy roof. I didn't go to any real-estate dealers because I knew they would try to force the wrong thing on me and make me horribly uncomfortable. I knew that when the destined moment came I should find my house. But it must be let alone, I thought, to happen by itself like a friendship or a love affair.

Nevertheless, I was sure that I saw it in my mind's eye very much as it would turn out to be. Unquestionably, for me, a very small childish spinster, it should be small, something mignonne and doll-like. I had thought of an old Cape Cod cottage with a trumpet vine, or a cluster of outbuildings on some old Topsfield or Ipswich farm—a creamhouse, cobbler's shop, and woodshed all fastened together by narrow passages and made into something fascinating and doll-size. I had once seen a house like that which its owner called The Thimbles because each building was no bigger than a thimble. After that, thimble was the word used by me and my family to describe the thing that was supposed to be suitable for me, for my size and my needs, and it was understood and approved by everybody that sooner or later I should find and buy myself a thimble. Therefore when I noticed the FOR SALE sign on a very large high square house on Penobscot Bay overlooking the Bagaduce River and the islands and the Cape Rozier hills, and when just out of casual curiosity I stepped inside to look at it, I was awestruck by the force of destiny. I didn't recognize this huge house at all. I had never seen it in my mind's eye. But I knew that whether I liked it or not this at last was my house. It frightened me very much. And filled me with astonishing joy, quite out of keeping with my size and my spinsterhood.

The owner's wife showed us over it and said she didn't know what price her husband was asking for it. My sister-in-law laughed scornfully at the idea of an unattached person like me in rather fragile health buying that enormous place. It would have been more suitable for her with her family of children. We all laughed heartily at the idea as we went roaming just for fun through those high square rooms. But I laughed with a secret terror and a secret exultation because I knew that I had met my fate. I did not tell them what I knew, however, and we stepped out of the house to all appearances as casually as we had stepped in. We thanked the woman and did not leave our names.

In spite of the fact that we did not leave our names, the pompous owner of the house came the next day to see me at my boarding-place. His wife, he said, had heard my companions call me Kitty while we were going through the house, and he had inquired everywhere until he found out who Kitty was and where she was staying. It happened that my brother and sister-in-law had gone home that morning and I was staying on alone until the end of the season. I was very thankful that they had gone when Fate called in person. It is much better that Fate should cleave its way without any futile protests except from the victim. It should be a clean-cut rendezvous à deux.

When the man told me the price of his house I thought he must be feeble-minded. But as he talked I saw that he felt contempt and hatred for the house and was not capable of understanding that it could have beauty or value for anyone. He had been trying for a long time, in his contemptuous way, to get rid of it. It had come into his possession through a business deal, and he and his wife had lived in it against their natures. They wanted a convenient little bungalow. They didn't like fireplaces. "I am not a fireplace man," he said, and his phrase fascinated me and puzzled me as I half listened to him.

My heart was beating very fast as I turned his unbelievable price over in my mind and for a few seconds I did not speak. He went on talking persuasively, evidently thinking my silence meant that his price had frightened me. "Why, the horse-chestnut tree alone is worth a thousand dollars. You couldn't buy it for that," he said. My awareness of destiny on the day before had seemed fantastic to me merely on the ground that such a fine old house would be hopelessly out of the reach of a person like me, whose great ambition had been to buy only a little weatherbeaten shed. Now the obstacle of money was miraculously swept away. The price was even much less than the money that I had to spend. I could not only buy the house but have enough money left over to make all the necessary changes.

When this man who was not a fireplace man was gone I knew that I must make a decision. I had never had any responsibility nor any business experience. I had never been out in the world at all, as they say. During the next few days I was in such a frightful torment that I wished I had never seen the house. It would have been so much easier to go on dreaming of a poetic little doll house. Reality is unbelievably terrifying after one has done nothing but dream.

In the daytime I saw the house as it had struck me so forcibly the first time—that is, as a promise of a new era for me, the starting point for a happier and more creative life than I had ever known. But in the middle of the night everything was reversed and I shook in my bed. It gave me a feeling of pure panic. Then I was ashamed of myself for even considering such a wild foolhardy thing. In the night

9

the house changed into a monster that was teasing me only to lead me into some sort of fiasco from which my family would have to rescue me. I was constantly comparing the value and authenticity of this night fear with my morning confidence.

Then when my mind seemed as thick as mud, stupefied by indecision, out of it like daredevil jonquils and crocuses would spring fragile shoots of joy connected with some detail I had thought of in imagining the future life of the house. It was the same exultant joy that I always used to feel when I was beginning to write a poem. My wrists ached with the delicious ache of creative desire.

So the prospect of buying that house gave me first one and then another of those two contradictory feelings. I discovered that my decision was only a question of whether I preferred to be governed by fear or by a creative feeling, and although I was very frightened I knew I could not choose fear. The panic terrors that came in the night might scare me half to death, but I would never let them decide things for me. Then and there I invented this rule for myself to be applied to every decision I might have to make in the future. I would sort out all the arguments and see which belonged to fear and which to creativeness, and other things being equal I would make the decision which had the larger number of creative reasons on its side. I think it must be a rule something like this that makes jonquils and crocuses come pushing through cold mud.

I went to a party where there was a fortuneteller reading palms. "You are going to take on a new responsibility very soon," she told me. "The result will be that your life will become much more interesting than it has been, and your health much better." This prophecy thrilled me through and through, like the first spoken declaration of a love which one has been only intuitively aware of until then. Still I hesitated, still deliciously hanging to the edge of the chasm. Perhaps I enjoyed that delicious agony while it lasted. It could only last a few days.

Then one evening, obsessed and indecisive still, and deeply excited, I was driving with someone, and I asked to go around the road where the house stood. I wanted to see how it looked at night. It was the last house on a dark little road that looped one end of the town. It faced a field with one end toward the road. A great horse-chestnut tree stood at the entrance where a brick path led from the road to the front door. Beyond and behind the house its fields fell away down to the tiny lighted windows and peaked roofs of Water Street, and to the harbor with its dark islands beyond. We came to the turn of the road that evening, and I saw my house facing me across the field. A yellow beam of light was shining from the fanlight over the door. That yellow beam was shining through the long white skirts of a fog, a heavy coast-of-Maine fog, the fresh dripping fog of those fir-scented islands and cold tidal rivers. For some reason, that moment was the decisive one. When I saw my benign, handsome old house that August night, wrapped in a thick Maine fog, I knew I could not wait another day.

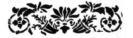

11

4

THUS begins the story of my house, with my erratic choice of one so different from the kind I had been thinking I must and certainly would have. It was like an amazingly unsuitable marriage, and as in the case of all unsuitable marriages there was a reason back of it, or it would never have happened. Before I go on with the adventures that followed immediately I must tell what that reason was. Since the story of my house is a story of the liberation of a human being, I must tell what it was that had made me a prisoner, and that made the simple act of buying a house so significant and exciting to me.

As far back as I can remember I have been fascinated by the marvelous transformations which take place when a very simple sort of magic is applied to things. Even the most everyday transformation of something undesirable into something desirable has, to me, a tremendous magic power back of it, and it is a power which I believe in using more deliberately and often than most people do. Everyone marvels at such transformations when they come by accident, but it never seems to occur to anyone to make them happen at will. I am shocked by the ignorance and wastefulness with which persons who should know better throw away the things they do not like. They throw away experiences, people, marriages, situations, all sorts of things because they do not like them. If you throw away a thing it is gone. Where you had something you have nothing. Your hands are empty, they have nothing to work on. Whereas, almost all those things which get thrown away are capable of being worked over by a little simple magic into just the opposite of what they were. So that in the place of something you detested you have something you can adore. And you have had the most thrilling kind of experience, because nothing is more thrilling than working the magic of transformation. The reason this kind of work seems to fall into the classification of magic is because it is so easy. It is not work at all. It is, simply, magic.

This trick of changing one thing into another thing is very well-known to us in fairy tales. We are almost born knowing about it, as if it were an instinctive part of us. Because we know it so well we are always on pins and needles when the hero or heroine forgets it in the thick of disaster, strangely forgets that he or she has the talisman which was given to be used in need—in just this very moment. Then when all seems lost—suddenly out of the pocket it comes, remembered in the nick of time, as you knew it would be, and behold! evil is changed into good, danger into safety, poverty to riches. The magic of transformation! Dearest of all these changes because it is the most intimate of them all is the change from physical ugliness to beauty. First there is the cruel imprisonment of the prince or princess in an ugly shape, and then the merciful counterpart of that cruelty, when the despised creature suddenly arises in his true shape, flawless and serene. In fairy stories the hero or heroine never fails to remember the magic solution before it is too late. But most human beings never remember at all that in almost every bad situation there is the possibility of a transformation by which the undesirable may be changed into the desirable.

The Little Locksmith

This is the story of such transformations, both large and small, and now in the beginning I will tell the nature of the predicament which first made this kind of magic dear to me—the predicament and the magic together which made necessary and possible at last my visit to the almond-shaped island which lay in the palm of my right hand. For of course, without a predicament, there is no need of magic.

When I was five years old I was changed from a rushing, laughing child into a bedridden, meditative one. As the years passed, my mother explained to me just what had happened, and why I had to lie so still. She told me how lucky I was that my parents were able to have me taken care of by a famous doctor. Because, without the treatment I was having, I would have had to grow up into a—well, I would have had to be, when I grew up, like the little locksmith who used to come to our house once in a while to fix locks. I knew the little locksmith, and after this, when he came, I stared at him with a very strange intimate feeling. He never looked back at me. His eyes were always down at what he was doing, and he apparently did not want to talk with or look at anybody. He was very fascinating indeed. He was not big enough to be considered a man, yet he was not a child. In the back his coat hung down from an enormous sort of peak, where the cloth was worn and shiny, between his shoulders, and he walked with a sort of bobbing motion. In front his chin was almost down on his chest, his hands were long, narrow, and delicate, and his fingers were much cleverer than most people's fingers. There was something about him, something that was indescribably alluring to a child. Because he was more like a gnome than a human being he naturally seemed to belong to our world more than to the grown-up world. Yet he seemed to refuse to belong to our world or anybody else's. He acted as if he lived all alone in a very private world of his own.

Somehow I knew that there was a special word that the grownups called a person shaped like the little locksmith, and I knew that to ordinary healthy grownups it was a terrible word. And the strange thing was that I, Katharine, the Butlers' darling little girl, had barely escaped that uncanny shape and that terrible word. Because I was being taken care of by a famous doctor nobody would ever guess, when I grew up, that I might have been just like the little locksmith. Staring wonderingly at him, *I* knew it. I knew that compared with him I was wonderfully lucky and safe. Yet deep within me I had a feeling that underneath my luck and safeness the real truth was that I really belonged with him, even if it was never going to show. I was secretly linked with him, and I felt a strong, childish, amorous pity and desire toward him, so that there was even a queer erotic charm for me about his gray shabby clothes, the strange awful peak in his back, and his cross, unapproachable sadness which made him not look at other people, not even at me lying on my bed and staring sideways at him.

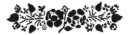

15

5

I WAS able to stare at him from my bed because I could turn my head from side to side. I had worn a bald spot as big as a quarter on the back of my head just from turning it to look at the people who were in the room with me, or turning it the other way to look out into the branches of the tulip tree that grew outside my window. For the doctor's treatment consisted in my being strapped down very tight on a stretcher, on a very hard sloping bed, with my shoulders pressed against a hard pad. My head was kept from sinking down on my chest like the little locksmith's by means of a leather halter attached to a rope which went through a pulley at the head of the bed. On the end of the rope hung a five-pound iron weight. This mechanism held me a prisoner for twenty-four hours a day, without the freedom to turn or twist my body or let my chin move out of its uptilted position in the leather halter, except to go from side to side. My back was supposed to be kept absolutely still.

I spent joyous days as most children do who are strapped into iron frames or pinned down on boards like specimen butterflies. The child who is denied his natural scope seems to develop a compensating activity on a microscopic scale. Everything small, everything near at hand, becomes magnified in its importance, and very dear and delightful to him. He gets untold pleasure out of things that ordinary people can hardly see at all.

Although my back was imprisoned, my hands and arms and mind were free. I held my pencil and pad of paper up in the air above my face, and I wrote microscopic letters and poems, and made little books of stories, and very tiny pictures. I sewed the smallest doll clothes anybody had ever seen, with the narrowest of hems and most delicious little ruffles. I painted with water colors and made paper dolls and dollhouse furniture out of paper. I loved paper, colored paper, fancy tissue, and crepe paper and ordinary white or brown paper too. The commonest substance in the world, it had for me an uncommon charm because of all the things it suggested to my mind that could be made out of it. I used to hold a piece of paper in my hands up above my face and let my eyes dwell on it in a sort of trance until, like the Japanese flowers, it would begin to bloom. Appearing on it, in my mind's eye, some little object would take shape which to me seemed the most adorable little object in the world—a house, a box, a fan, or a screen. Then, having seen the image of it, I would put my scissors and paints and paste and fingers to work in order to bring that darling little object into being. It was surely the magic of transformation in this performance that made it so delightful, and almost awe-inspiring. Paper was the nearest thing to nothing in the way of material, and yet it was possible to make it into something that people would exclaim over and fall in love with— something that had a shape, something that opened and shut or stood up. It was something precious made out of nothing.

When my hands and arms grew tired from this close application I had my treasures to enjoy. These were numerous little objects that I loved. They were always near me, on the table beside my bed. There

17

was my Revolutionary bullet, for instance, which one of my cousins had found in the cellar of an old house. I have no idea why I was so devoted to my bullet, except that it was interesting to feel of and to hold. It was round, and piercingly heavy in the palm of my hand in comparison to its small size, and it had a rough uneven surface, doubtless from having been turned out in haste by the rebels. To me, it had great character and importance. So much so, that with that completely idiotic disregard of appropriateness which 'children so often display I made a little embroidered velvet bag to keep it in, marked H. R. H. Bullet.

There was my gun-metal pencil, which somebody brought me from Paris. That, also, was most interesting to take hold of, because of its important-feeling weight in contrast to its size and compactness. It was like some valuable little instrument, rather than a mere pencil. It was a gun-metal cylinder with a brass ring in one end for a ribbon to go through, and it had three round imitation jewels, a ruby, a sapphire, and a pearl, in stubby gilt settings, which slid up and down in slits on its three sides. I pushed the ruby up the slit and out of the open end of the cylinder came a brass pencil that held a red lead. I pushed up the sapphire and the pencil with a blue lead appeared, or the pearl which held a black lead. Precious adorable thing, where are you gone, lost for so long?

Then I remember my Japanese rabbit. He was about one inch long, made of pottery, and covered with a warm gray glaze. He was hunched up into a little ball, his nose on the ground and his ears up against his back, the most compact and lovable little shape I ever saw. I liked rolling him around in the palm of my hand, then shutting my hand and hugging him tight. I would pretend he was only a pebble. When he was shut up in my hand he felt enough like one to fool anybody. Then I would open my fingers and give myself the surprise and joy of discovering that he was not a pebble at all, but a marvelous little rabbit. All over again as if I had never seen him before, I would study him and dote upon the perfect microscopic carving of his ears, eyes, nose, and whiskers.

I had a great many other Japanese things, too, thanks to Professor Morse. As I lay on my bed during my childhood I heard people talking about Japan a great deal, as if it were a newly discovered country. Professor Morse had just come back to Salem after living in Japan for many years, and I used to hear him excitedly telling my grandfather about all the things he had seen and learned there. I heard all the different grownups repeating to each other things he had told them about Japan and Japanese ways, telling about the prints and the pottery and the screens and the paper windows. More and more Japanese things kept coming into our house, and many of them came to me to use—such as rice paper, bamboo-handled paintbrushes, and bowls, and fragrant little wooden boxes. I held them in my hands, I felt them and smelled them. That fragrance! How it clung to each thing, as if it were the signature of Japan! I snuffed it in the pages of the folding books that were made of crepe paper as soft and crushable as thick silk; it was in the prints of terrible warriors and pale-faced women, and on the little pottery figures and the chopsticks; and most of all, perhaps,

19

that sharp fragrance filled all the smooth surfaces and every crack and corner of the softly shutting little wooden boxes.

Instead of the bright colors we were accustomed to, the colors the Japanese used were subtle tones of gray and brown. These mouselike colors were as surprising as a sudden hush in a place where everybody has been shouting. They were very humble colors, the ones we ignored and despised in our own paintboxes; and that they should be chosen as favorites, as they apparently were by the Japanese people, gave them a new mysterious importance, like a code language, in which a great deal of extra meaning is packed into plain ordinary words. In fact, this delight in modesty and humbleness, so foreign to us, which marked all Japanese things, seemed to hold a secret, a hidden message that we could not fully understand. I was not the kind of a child who ever paid any attention to grown-up learned talk. So Professor Morse's elucidation of the Japanese culture and view of life expressed by these objects went in one ear and out the other. Indeed, I was so much opposed to any troublesome mental effort that I doubt if it even came in one ear. But all my other senses were busy receiving with voluptuous joy the new experiences these objects gave me.

Because I was not able to explore and find for myself all the touching and tasting and feeling adventures that well children do as they dart on foot in every direction, I was quick to catch and cling tight to every interesting thing that came within reach of my bed, like the cannibalistic flowers that catch their food as it goes floating by. So I am grateful that Professor Morse brought treasures from

Japan to our neighborhood in Salem in the nineties while I was lying there very eager and still, and that my parents in their turn brought some of the treasures to my bed for me to hold and smell until they became almost a part of me.

Besides all my treasures, of course I had certain books always near me. I had my Boutet de Monvel books which I could live in for hours, staring for a long, long time at each illustrated page, soaking up into my brain and fingers for my own future use Boutet de Monvel's way of drawing certain things. I had books of pictures for gazing at and books of stories for reading, each one a different world I lived in—*Little Women, The Counterpane Fairy, Heidi, Cranford, Alice, The Cuckoo Clock, The Child's Garden of Verses, Lorna Doone, Don Quixote.* I read also the diary of Marie Bashkirtsev, *Rab and His Friends,* and Marjorie Fleming, Dickens' and Sir Walter Scott's novels, and Shakespeare. I had the *St. Nicholas Magazine* which came every month, causing wild eagerness and excitement and utter satisfaction in me and my brothers. We all contributed to the St. Nicholas League, and saw our verses and drawings printed, and won gold and silver badges. There were European children in the League, as well as Americans, and through the Letter Box I began a correspondence with a Swiss girl older than myself, Yvonne Jequier. I had admired her drawings in the League because they were so expert and had a different air from the ones made by American children. Her first letter in reply to mine awed me because it was written with a gracious courteousness that sounded more like a grown-up person than a child. I read it over and over, very

21

flattered at being addressed in such a style, and thrilled by her sweetness and good humor in carefully answering each question I had asked her about her life in the Alps, and making sympathetic and interested comments on everything that I had told her about myself. And most flattering of all, she enclosed one of her own drawings.

For companions near at hand I had my brothers, Fergus and Warren, just older than I, and my little sister, Lurana, who was very cute to draw, and docile about posing for me. We were all made of the same stuff. The boys and I were a league, ourselves —especially Warren and I. I can never forget, for instance, the day when Warren showed me that there was more than one way to draw feet. I was like the Egyptians, I had not advanced beyond the practice of always making the feet exactly alike. I made them pointed flat away from each other. Suddenly Warren crept up to me and showed me a great secret about drawing feet, which burst upon me like the dawn of a new scientific truth. After that I always did them the new way—one foot pointing straight toward me and the other pointing daintily sideways—until another great day came when I noticed and imitated the wonderful feet in Boutet de Monvel's drawings. Another event of importance was the time when I made the stupendous discovery that brown and purple look the same by gaslight. One evening I was coloring a paper doll, and I asked to be allowed to finish it even though the gas had been lighted and it was time for me to stop. It was all done except the hair. I was allowed to finish it, and I painted the hair brown. The next morning I looked at my paper doll, and found that her hair was

22

purple. The boys and I were thunderstruck by this discovery, and it reverberated among us for years. After that, whenever we kept on painting after the lights were lit, we looked up and solemnly cautioned each other about brown and purple, like railroad engineers warning each other about foggy conditions and faulty signals.

Sometimes other children came to play with us, but they were all rather dim. They came into my room and stood around heavily and watched what we were doing. But they didn't have gumption or imagination enough to join us in the things we liked to do. All they could understand were games like tag and hide-and-seek, and if my brothers were absorbed in more subtle occupations up in my room these visitors would have to stand around and wait. And when finally the boys rose up and went galloping through the house or out of doors to play active games, and my little sister went rushing after them, I never felt a pang as might have been expected, nor any sense of being left behind. I must have known that I could always call them back by writing a new poem or drawing a new picture, and they would come eagerly to see it. There was no need for me to feel sad because we all so wholeheartedly took it for granted that no other amusement was really interesting compared with drawing or writing or making something. It seemed as if I were the lucky one because I could do these things all day long and never be interrupted by having somebody tell me to pick up my clothes or start for school. I was exempt from all the drudgery the others had to go through every day, and my room was like a busy studio—the natural center of the house for the others. And when they were not there I was never lonely because I always had my nurse to talk to and order about.

When strange children came into the room there would sometimes be one among them who took a ghoulish pleasure in staring at my halter and rope and whispering about it to the child next to him. Even without looking up, my brothers and I knew when this happened and it filled us with fury, with disgust and contempt for the child's stupidity in not knowing what was important and what was not important. The first time it happened it produced a very surprising sensation in me about myself, which was like tasting a queer new taste that I didn't know existed. Something repulsive had come into my room, something that surely had nothing to do with me. Yet the strange part of it was that the child's staring eyes said that it had everything to do with me, they said that the repulsive thing was myself and my halter and rope. As soon as I recovered from the first shock of it I knew that the child's eyes lied. I had been told that my name, Katharine, meant crystal, clear—from a Greek word, katharsis. And I felt inside myself, as part of me, a crystal quality, a sort of happiness that was like a spring always bubbling fresh and new. No matter if I tried I could never, inside myself, feel anything except happy and sparkling. It was constitutionally impossible for me to feel that any part of me was repulsive. So when that presence came into my room again, and always with certain children, I knew it was something which was really a part of them more than a part of me. But I could not help tasting again that queer astonished sensation about myself whenever they stared at me in that particular way of theirs which made some-

24

thing loathsome and fascinating out of me and the paraphernalia of my cure.

This same feeling of my own intrinsic separateness was always with me, too, when certain grownup callers insisted on coming burblingly upstairs "to see poor little Katharine." I could always hear them coming and I knew just what to expect. I didn't need to be very subtle to realize from their puffing exclamations of pity and their heavily tactful asides that these visitors imagined that I was unfortunate. Under their breath I heard the gruesome word "afflicted." Such people bored me beyond words. They didn't seem like real living people. I knew they were not interested in me at all as Katharine, only as "poor little Katharine." They never paid any attention to what I was drawing or making, they were blind to all the interesting treasures around me. They were not real people, surely, but just large meaningless objects that had got into my room by mistake and were very much in the way there. Ignoring everything under their noses which would have interested them if they had been alive, they could only seem to see the one thing in the room which was not interesting and not important except that it was doing me good, my halter and rope. And they would stand staring and asking questions and boring me with their stupid pity until my mother or my nurse finally led them away. The only impression, luckily, that was left on me by these visitors was disgust for their ignorance and a fresher satisfaction in my own affairs.

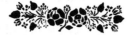

6

AS far as I knew from personal experience those boring old lady visitors of mine and the children who sometimes came and stared at me were the most disturbing sort of persons the world contained. We had no volcanoes in our family. Consequently there were no eruptions of anger or jealousy or selfishness. I knew from hearsay and from reading that these emotions existed and that they were shocking hideous things, but they never came into our midst to disturb our peace and friendliness toward each other. We gave things back and forth to each other as a matter of course. Brothers and sisters who fought to get things away from each other seemed to us incredibly stupid and vulgar. What fun did they have? We were always so busy and interested making things and doing things together that the passions of ownership and competition never had a chance to grow in us. From this mature sort of childhood we grew up, as may be imagined, very immature and ignorant emotionally, and not very well prepared to understand more violent people when we met them later on.

Our parents had preserved our ignorance by their own dignity and reserve which made them hide their own emotional life away from us completely. I should never have guessed that they had any life different and apart from ours if it had not been for two or three mysterious pieces of evidence that came to me by accident—once, a half-overheard fragment of a strange sentence—once, the terrible sound of a man crying—and once a single cry of despair or grief from my mother in another room, followed by a quickly shut door and then silence. These sounds, suddenly breaking in on my peculiarly protected, tranquil, and impersonal life were as startling as the sudden, unexplained appearance of blood. I shook when I heard them, with sudden emotion aroused by something I did not even know about. I did not want to know what it was. I shrank from it. I was afraid, because whatever it was I had a feeling that it was too big for me to bear, or even to know existed. I had my own cosmic troubles that were too big for me, but they were somehow a part of me. There was a sound, a timbre, in human troubles that I could not endure at all. My world, mostly inanimate, and myself, immovable, were not geared for those troubles and emotions.

There was, however, one poignant emotion to which we had all been awakened by the sensitiveness of our parents, and which we all enjoyed consciously. This was an awareness of something which I cannot describe, because its peculiar quality lay in its being indescribable. I can only call it the ineffable charm of life. We were sensitive to the atmosphere of certain times and places, of certain unpredictable external things, which gave us an acute pleasure which we all seemed to feel and understand in each other. There was not too much stress laid upon this experience. It was felt much more than it was talked about. It was a feeling of ecstasy that was almost distress when it came, because it came so bound up and clogged by our own stupid feeling—the stupid ache of never being able to equal it or match it with anything like itself when it came.

There was one favorite experience which above

all others gave us that feeling. That was our annual coming-home—from Stowe. Stowe was the village in northern Vermont where we spent every summer in a little farmhouse that had belonged to our grandparents. When the last day came we said passionate good-bys to everything, and leaving that world of mountain coolness and resinous clear air we traveled all day in the train, arriving at last in the city in the dusk of a hot fall night. Then it began to come, that indescribable feeling, a spirit that moved in us, violently and strangely—a sweet and intense awareness of the drama and wonder of life, produced in us by that change of scene.

We loved Vermont and Stowe with a passionate love, and yet on that evening our new, poignant memory of it made us love the city in no ordinary way. The September mountain air that we had breathed that very morning made our sudden entrance into the evening city strangely thrilling to us, and the September city heat came over us with a wonderful languorousness.

When I traveled, in those days, I had to be carried on my stretcher, and I was brought up from the station laid across the two seats of an old-fashioned cab. It was a short drive up from the station, and it was with that drive that the best of it began, for me at least. The dark swaying plumes of the elm trees overhead in the almost tropical twilight, the clop-clop of the horse's feet on the city pavement, the queer smell of the inside of the cab, were inexpressibly beautiful to me.

We reached our little Victorian house and saw again in the half-dark the fancy iron fence along the front of our garden, the brick walk going to the side door, and the trellised arch over the walk where the great sumptuous trumpet vine grew. I was carried through the gate and along the brick walk, my fingers clinging tight to the slender iron framework of my stretcher as I went swaying forward to the uneven rhythm of my nurse's and my father's footsteps, one at each end of me.

During that brief passage I smelled again the burned, dusty, Septembery smell of the city garden, and heard again how the air was all filled with the mysterious shrill ringing of the September crickets. I went under the dark bower of the trumpet vine that I loved. Its rich, extravagant summer growth, the long sprays that hung out of it and moved with every breath of air, and the burnt orange of the slender tube-shaped flowers made something for me as uncommunicable as a remembered song. It was that great rich trumpet vine, especially the trumpet vine, that gave, to me, at least, the feeling of ineffable mystery and charm that was always and eternally a part of that night when we came home from Stowe.

The boys had of course walked up from the station and got there long before us and would already have explored the garden. And Warren, slipping past me as I was being maneuvered into the house, would perhaps drop a bunch of grapes into the nest between my ear and my shoulder. I could smell them and feel them against my neck, our little dark-blue Salem grapes that grew in the arbor at the very back of our garden. Or perhaps Fergus would drop on my chest a moist and beautiful autumn rose from the rose garden on the terrace. So in ecstasy I went sailing through the side door and up the back stairs, my stretcher hoisted and quivering and almost perpendicular until I arrived at last in my old room and was moored again to my bed beside the tulip tree.

My nurse, unstrapping me from my stretcher and rolling me back and forth to get my arms out of my sleeves, would take off my traveling clothes and put my thinnest nightgown on me for the hot city night. I lay and watched her and listened to her in a kind of delicious hypnotism—her hand reaching up and pulling down the window shades, and the look of her back as she opened bureau drawers, and the rustly sounds she made as she began to put things away. Every little action, every little touch and sound, was different that night, and wonderful.

We lay awake as long as we could manage to stay awake, all four of us, in our different rooms—half conscious, inarticulate, impressionable, stupid children—so that we might enjoy to the full our queer annual rapture of hearing over and over the slow rise and fall of the Salem crickets' trill, and the strange, familiar sound of people's feet going up and down on the brick sidewalk in the street, and of staring dreamily at our strange familiar bedroom walls and watching the way the city arc light made great moving shadows of horse-chestnut leaves and branches.

After the first night at home that particular magic began to fade and was soon all gone, locked away somewhere in a cupboard of time, precious and strange, to wait for our little lives to live another enormous year around again. After that night Salem was just Salem, and Stowe became the word that always could evoke for us something marvelous and far away.

For me, that one night was a blessed reprieve, because it drugged me with new sensations strong enough to make me forget for a few hours a secret that weighed on me eternally. For although my daytime life was so delightful and absorbing, when evening came, I left it and descended into hell.

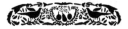

7

I HAD two hideous familiars, two fiendish jailers, who with the sudden onrush of darkness and solitude leapt on me every night and seized me one on each side and would not let me go. These two were two Awful Thoughts which my mind had hit upon in its childish explorings and had been poisoned by and made sick and swollen by, as if one of them had been a snake that had bitten me and the other an evil plant that had stung me. One of the two Awful Thoughts was the endlessness of Space, and the other was the endlessness of Time. Every night, held in the grip of these two horrors, my little brain rolled over backward in humble, piteous convulsions of fear, and my body trembled and shook with the hideous disaster of having been born into this awful universe, of being forced to exist in the very arms of these two unthinkable things.

Yet, on the other hand, *not* to have been born, never to have been me at all, to have remained forever nonexistent somewhere in outer Space was even more lonely and terrible to think of. There was no escape from thinking, in life or in death, since I believed in the immortality of my own consciousness —that it was doomed to continue *forever* either in heaven or in hell. Each night the whole terrible realization would spread slowly and surely to the very edges of my body and mind, soaking me, cooking me, in the pure poison of horror. Like a terrified mouse, my mind would scurry this way and that for a hole to hide in, for some little nest that I could curl up in. But there was no such little hole. All the daytime life and its thoughts which I loved so much became at night suddenly unreliable and false. My cousins, our jokes, Christmas presents, my dolls, the Woodsey Path in Stowe, my birthday and what I wanted, the *St. Nicholas*—I ran appealing and stricken among them all—my nicest, dearest, daytime thoughts—and they availed nothing against the feeling of cosmic loneliness and doom. My awful thoughts breathed an icy breath on all the charm and fun and adorableness of the life of day and made it crumple into nothing, and prove itself to have been no more than a pitiful deception. Every night I looked backward upon my darling little cheerful loves and occupations of the day just passed, like a mother torn from her children.

Every night, as if I were compelled as a sort of punishment, I went over and over the same hopeless path, climbing up to the brink of unthinkableness and then tumbling back again, up and back, up and back—until I could actually feel the aching groove the repetition made inside my head. Every night I would endure and endure and endure, knowing I must not call or cry out until I simply could not bear it any longer. When the unbearable limit suddenly came, I screamed, I called, Papa! Then I listened, boiling with fear. It was worse to have screamed if nobody came—more horrible, more lonely. Sometimes nobody heard me the first time, and I called again. Papa! . . . Then, oh, merciful! I heard footsteps—slow, calm, cozy footsteps. Into the back hall, up the stairs, across the threshold of my room, the footsteps brought my tall, narrow-shouldered, frail Papa.

He sat down close beside me, and put his healing and comforting hand upon me. Wonderful hand! . . . Wonderful calm quietness! . . . Then he began to recite Wordsworth's poem about the daffodils. After that, Lochinvar. Always the same two poems. Then perhaps he would sit without speaking, and in the calm loving stillness that he created between us I was supposed to lose my childish nervous fears and begin to grow sleepy. But even while he sat so close to me in the darkness we were separated. For I was sure that he had never thought about endlessness. Otherwise he could not have been so calm. He, like all the other strangely casual grownups, had apparently never come across these Awful Thoughts. His innocent mind had never explored as far as mine had done. He, like the rest, could be so preoccupied with the cozy life of our earth, of our sitting room downstairs, of his books, of the new *Atlantic Monthly*, that he was unbelievably forgetful of the awful abyss in which our earth was hanging.

Like someone trying again and again to fling himself over a wall that is just too high, I kept trying in spite of my failure every night to bring myself to the fearful point of speaking of it to him. I would work myself up by a terrific force of will to a decision to ease my mind come what would; I got my first sentence up to the threshold of possible plausible utterance and at last a few parched dreadful words would cross my lips. Then my heart thundered as I paused to see what the effect would be. My father, to my amazement, remained perfectly unperturbed. "Let's think about Stowe," he would say. "See if you can see the Woodsey Path in your mind's eye. Tell me, can you see how it looks when the raspberries are ripe on the wild raspberry bushes?" Tears of disappointment rushed to my eyes in the darkness. He didn't know! He couldn't understand! To please him, I would try to force myself to think about the raspberry bushes or whatever else he suggested to soothe me, while I gave up once more the hope of ever sharing my suffering. The contrast between my horrors and his simple unquestioning innocence and tranquillity was too much for me. I felt as if I were the mature person and he the happy unconscious child. And so I felt a yearning tenderness and pity for him, and an even more lonely despair for myself.

I realized again and again that grownups were too cheerful, even the sensitive ones like my father, to understand really terrible things. Even if the horror is unescapably true, as it seemed to me to be, the grownups cannot see its truth, cannot grasp it, because it is too foreign to their easy comfortable way of thinking. The very calmness that grownups seem to bring with them into the fear-crowded darkness of a child's bedroom too often consists only in a hopeless insulation and imperviousness on their part, making them seem so superior and panic-proof that the child is driven to conceal from them all the really queer and terrible things he thinks or feels.

34

I myself often wondered, even then, if many of these imperturbable grownups would have been able to stand the continuous relentless mental suffering that I was having every night.

In my mental loneliness I thought that I had been initiated by chance into a knowledge that no human being was supposed to have or endure, and certainly no child. Because of it, I felt myself secretly an exile from the happy unconscious level of existence that my father and everyone else that I knew inhabited. I was banished and damned forever. It was as if they breathed a different air from me. I contemplated my situation with a fearful wistfulness, because I could see so well how blissfully happy I would have been, with my talents, and all my treasures, *St. Nicholas,* our summers in beloved Stowe, the grape arbor, the playhouse, if only I could wipe out forever that unlucky day when my mind had roamed too far. Such was the underlying sense of cosmic woe and cosmic disaster that curdled the joy of my childhood. And all the while some docile unconscious sweetness kept me from ever questioning the disaster that had befallen my body.

It is a very long time now since I lay quaking on my bed and my father sat beside me night after night, so tenderly aware of me, and never knew that I was in hell. Now that I am grown up myself I have become strangely casual and calm about the universe and I can tell it at last. But it is many years too late, he is gone, long, long ago—and it doesn't matter any more. And too late I know that his tranquillity those evenings concealed from me agonies of his own that were almost as bad as mine. Why couldn't we both have cried out and told each other all about our horrors and clung together and really known each other, father and child?

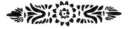

8

WHEN I was fifteen this horizontal life of night and day was ended. In that year I was pronounced cured; I was to get up at last and see things from a perpendicular and movable point of view, after watching them for so long from a horizontal and fixed one. Everything would look different, of course. Also, I knew that I myself would look different standing up from the way I had looked lying down. Why, at the great age of fifteen I didn't even know how tall I was! And I had begun to wonder secretly about my back. There was that unknown territory between my shoulders where the tuberculosis had lodged and burrowed for so long. How much it had disfigured me I didn't know. As I had grown older there had been a baffling silence in regard to that side of my illness, and I never dared to ask. Nobody guessed that I was secretly worrying about it, and I could not tell them. Nobody guessed, because, I suppose, I gave the impression of being such a happy, humorous child. But when I was alone in the room I sometimes slid my hand up under me to explore that fateful part. But my hand always got strangely panic-stricken and came hurrying back without making me any wiser than before. My hand seemed to be mortally afraid of that place, which remained therefore unknown, waiting for the day when I should get up and stand plainly revealed.

Although my mother had so often told me, when I was little, how lucky I was, as I grew older she never spoke of my being lucky. Instead, quite a different feeling seemed to come over her whenever she or anybody else spoke of my "trouble" as it was called. I must first explain that when I was young my mother seemed to me dull and uninteresting compared with my father. He and I were conscious of each other, almost as lovers are. Everything he said held my attention, and was interesting and essential to me. In comparison, my mother seemed to have to think and talk about a lot of unessential things, and her real self, for me, was swamped and obscured by them. I had a feeling that she didn't like unessential things, but that she didn't quite know how to manage them easily and get them out of the way. So she labored awkwardly, directing the house and servants, and she worried, and had to go to bed with sick headaches. Sometimes I felt very maternal toward her, she had such a hard time doing things that I thought looked quite easy. My own hands were so much more skillful than hers, for instance, that if she tried to make a paper doll for me she seemed to me like a clumsy younger child. She was not an artist, or a craftsman, like the rest of us, and so she thought we were much more wonderful than we were. I never saw her eyes really shine with happiness as much as they did when she was admiring us as artists, and treasuring all the things we made. Then she made herself, in comparison, seem humble and unimportant. In matters of our conduct as human beings she was relentless,

37

and we feared her as we feared God. We learned very young to be good and to obey and to respect our father and mother. But when she was admiring us as artists she gave us a feeling of absolute freedom from authority. We were all for weighing and criticizing each other's works. We knew to a hair's breadth which was better than another, and why. But she liked everything we did, our good things and also the ones we would have torn up and thrown away. She gathered them all together and kept and treasured them, and her eyes shone over us with a pride and a tenderness that I shall never see again.

Because of this humble uncritical attitude of hers toward art, I didn't notice her very much, and when I did I often wished that she were more exciting and knew how to do things herself. But once in a great while, when somebody spoke of my illness or she mentioned it herself, she was all changed. I couldn't very well not notice her then. A terrific wave of pain sprang up in her blue eyes, and it was evident suddenly that the pain was always there, controlled, inside her, like something terribly alive, always ready to leap up and hurt her all over again. She never cried, but her self-control was worse than crying.

"I ought never to have *let* it happen! It was wicked! Wicked!" she would burst out. And then, immediately after, I witnessed the silent and to me awful struggle as for some reason she fought against the physical symptoms of her grief. Not a tear ever succeeded in getting past the barrier of her will, and not a sob. But during those few seconds when she could not trust herself to speak, and her gentian-blue eyes were fiercely widened to prevent the tears

38

from coming into them as she stared away from me, out of the window, anywhere, away from me, and swallowed back that great lump of sadness and forced it away down into the secret part of her being, I was awe-struck and shaken, much more than I would have been to see her yield to tears. Her secretive Spartan way made crying seem like an enemy that one must never submit to. The awesome struggle that it cost her affected me almost as if I had been forced to watch her from a distance struggling all alone with a savage animal and managing by sheer force of her will and character to keep it at bay.

When she was like that I could not very well not notice her or think she was uninteresting. Then her aliveness frightened me. And I loved her more than I could possibly have told. I felt a furious will to cherish her and protect her and never to let her suffer, when I got old enough to influence or control her. Yet I could not show her what I felt. Besides being inarticulate myself, I knew that I had seen something in her that she thought I was too young to see or even to know about, and I knew I must pretend I hadn't seen it. It was not her concern for me that made me love her so much then. It was because I saw her in the grip of essential things, and she became alive and fiery and very brave. I felt humble before her, for myself and for all the rest of us toward whom she had made herself seem unclever and unimportant.

Although I felt an almost unbearable tenderness and love for her in those moments, I felt hatred and rebellion too. I hated and rejected the idea that there was anything tragic about my illness, or that she was to blame. I was angry because when she battled with those terrible surging tears I had to battle too. Watching her, I felt a violent emotion suddenly throbbing against my throat, surging and aching in my chest. For she seemed to waken something in me that was a disgusting traitor to my conscious self, a sorrow over my own plight that leaped up out of the depth of me, and answered her with a grieving that seemed to understand and match her own. I could love her piteous sorrow for me, but I loathed and despised it in myself. And I pushed it away from me with an almost masculine strength and confidence in my own soundness and well-being. This rebellion made me appear hard and cold toward her, just at the moment when I loved her most.

Yet I always longed to know intimately and adore and caress that real fiery self of hers. Why did she hide it from her children and almost from herself? It seemed as if she thought that if she ever once let her emotion escape from under her control its poignancy would be unbearable, and would destroy her and destroy us all. Whatever the reason, when these moments arrived they passed in fierce silence and aloofness. The hearts of the mother and the child ached in pity for each other, each separate, stoical, and alone.

So, lying still and watching her, I was tense and fighting for her, helping her with all my might not to be overcome by the enemy that was trying to make us both cry and break out into sobs. I knew that if anything could make her lose the battle it would be to have me be anything except the happy unconscious child she thought I was. And besides, except when she acted like this, I *was* happy. After all, what was there so sad about me and my illness? It was a mystery to me. I thought my mother's sadness must be just a phenomenon of mother love, which exaggerates everything.

When I got up at last, fifteen years old, and had learned to walk again, one day I took a hand glass and went to a long mirror to look at myself, and I went alone. I didn't want anyone, my mother least of all, to know how I felt when I saw myself for the first time. But there was no noise, no outcry; I didn't scream with rage when I saw myself. I just felt numb. That person in the mirror *couldn't* be me. I felt inside like a healthy, ordinary, lucky person— oh, not like the one in the mirror! Yet when I turned my face to the mirror there were my own eyes looking back, hot with shame. I had turned out after all, like the little locksmith—oh, not so bad, nearly—but enough like the little locksmith to be called by that same word.

What I felt that day did not fit in with the pleasant cheerful atmosphere of our family, any more than my horrors had fitted in. There was no place for it among us. It was something in another language. It was in the same language as my mother's suppressed panic-stricken grief, and I would have died rather than let that come to the surface of our cheerful life, for her to see and endure in me. And so from that first moment, when I did not cry or make any sound, it became impossible that I should speak of it to anyone, and the confusion and the panic of my discovery were locked inside me then and there, to be faced alone, for a very long time to come.

Here then was the beginning of my predicament.

41

A hideous disguise had been cast over me, as if by a wicked stepmother. And I now had ahead of me, although I didn't know it, the long, blind, wistful struggle of the fairy tales. I had to wander stupidly and blindly, searching for I didn't know what, following fantastically wrong clues, until at last I might hit upon a magic that could set me free.

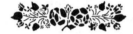

9

AT the very beginning it was lucky for me that I found my brother Warren. Three things had ended suddenly all at the same time—my illness and my childhood and my father's life. When one thing ends another must begin. As I have already written, at the end of my illness there began my ignorant and lonely struggle to adapt myself to what I had seen in the mirror. At this same time my childhood ended and a thrilling ferment of new consciousness had begun to go on inside me which made me feel myself turning wonderfully into a haughty and grand young lady. Although my body was impeded in its growth and I was bewildered by its misfortune, my mind was not impeded. My mind grew independently of my body and independently of the shape of my body. It grew and behaved at first as if nothing were wrong with me anywhere. I was even more concerned at first with extricating myself from the disgrace of being considered a child than I was concerned with the fearful fact of my deformity. Now that I was up and walking around at last, like the rest of the world, I seemed to feel a fierce revenge against my bed and my invalid life, and especially against the bright little girl who had accepted it all so sweetly and submissively. I suddenly hated my adorable microscopic world, and all the little arts out of which with painstaking care I had constructed my joys. I hated the loving admiration of the grownups for me and everything I did. I felt fierce and rebellious and strong and mad toward them and myself. Something new had come into my mind, and it was like a labor agitator who furiously tries to destroy the docile contentment of workers who have so long adapted themselves to a narrow life that they do not even realize it is narrow. Out of loyalty to the new values that were dawning in me and making me, as I believed, into an entirely new person, I had to do cruel violence to the contented little girl. I had to emphasize my separateness from her in every possible way because the grownups persisted in clinging to her with an absurd devotion and insisting she was me. Whereas I knew with every part of myself that she was not me any more. I was through with her. I was through because a wonderful thing had happened to me. I had found suddenly that I was not frightened any more by the abstract ideas that had frightened the little girl so terribly in her bed. I had begun to fall at first gingerly and then boldly in love with the mystery of the Universe. Instead of wanting to curl my mind up and tuck it away in some cozy little place where it could never think those terrifying thoughts of death and birth and time, my mind suddenly wanted to reach out and embrace fearlessly those mysteries and become a conscious, proud part of them. It seemed to me that I had suddenly grown so tall that my head was among the stars. Relieved, by some miracle, of my cosmic fears, I felt an almost drunken sense of liberation, as if I had been released from a most abject slavery and admitted to the free and fearless aristocracy of the mind.

At this crucial time my father died, and on the day I lost him, after a long illness that had made him grow remote from me, I found my brother Warren. We sat side by side on the piazza of our house on the strange April morning when we became fatherless. We watched the undertakers coming up the steps into the house, and going busily back and forth between the house and their terrible high black carriage. I felt cruelly little sorrow, considering how very deeply my father had cherished and loved me, perhaps because his cultivating love had helped to create the little girl whom I was now intent on destroying. Instead, his death gave me an exultant happiness because it strengthened and intensified my new awareness and adoration of cosmic things. It made me feel mature and experienced and proud because I could see it in the radiance of the new daybreak that was in my mind. Death was another of the great and ordered mysteries of life, and, being so, it could never frighten me any more. In that revelation there was indescribable ecstasy and joy for the young mystic who was beginning to inhabit my mind and look out of my eyes.

Like every fifteen-year-old person, my mind was so new to thought, and I was consequently so naïve, that I examined everything that came before me with the feeling that it was an entirely new phenomenon and had never been examined by anybody before. And when I was struck that morning as we sat on the piazza by the thought that the noble mystery of death ought not to be intruded upon and degraded by these loathsome undertakers—officious, practical, busy little men like black ants running to and fro—I was thrilled and surprised by my own angry resentment. In my experience older people seemed to take everything for granted, and when I found that I did not take the undertakers for granted it also dawned on me that I must be a wild and revolutionary thinker. I thought I had hit upon a point of view that probably nobody else in the world had ever held before. It was a purifying, beautiful, joyous sensation of anger that I felt, and I knew for the first time that I could feel passionately about an idea. Something had blazed in me, and from the blaze I discovered a new element in myself, a combustible something that would always blaze again in defense of the mystery and sacredness in things, and against the queer, blind, blaspheming streak in human nature which instead of adoring, must vulgarize and exploit and insult life.

In my excitement I turned to my brother and burst out with some incoherent exclamation about how I hated the undertakers. To my astonishment he said that he knew how I felt, and that he hated them too. This was the first time that I had ever exchanged anything like an abstract idea with anyone, and I could feel my new self expand still more.

So my brother and I looked at each other that day with curiosity and surprise and each recognized in the other a new and unexpected friend. We had both deserted the two absorbed and happy children we had lately been, and in doing so we had lost each other. It was lucky for me that we met again at that moment, which, for me, would have been intolerably bewildering alone. We were just entering the period which is like a magic forest, into which nobody either older or younger than ourselves could possibly be admitted. We needed to escape from them, from all the others, because our turn had come. It was our precious turn to believe, deluded and untested as we were, that we and our generation were the elect— the only beings on earth whose vision of life was really pure and abstract, a mystic's vision. We had not yet allowed ourselves to be corrupted by any such despicable things as expediency or money. Our actions and plans were not yet crippled by any of the loathsome timidities and misrepresentations of common sense, or stifled altogether by the paralyzing fears by which children and old people are all degraded. From that time of awakening onward there was a wild enchantment crying and singing in my blood, the enchantment and excitement that come, by rights, with the flowering of the young human body and its short-lived perfection. My youthful singing blood did not seem to know the crazy fact that my body had stumbled against, and never could listen to it and learn it and take it in. My very joyous blood took it for granted that my body was unfolding simultaneously with my consciousness, and the song of my blood was so much a part of me that I forgot, over and over, and took it for granted too.

Over and over I forgot what I had seen in the mirror. It could not penetrate into the interior of my mind and become an integral part of me. I felt as if it had nothing to do with me; it was only a disguise.

But it was not the kind of disguise which is put on voluntarily by the person who wears it, and which is intended to confuse other people as to one's identity. My disguise had been put on me without my consent or knowledge like the ones in fairy tales, and it was I myself who was confused by it, as to my own identity. I looked in the mirror, and was horror-struck because I did not recognize myself. In the place where I was standing, with that persistent romantic elation in me, as if I were a favored fortunate person to whom everything was possible, I saw a stranger, a little, pitiable, hideous figure, and a face that became, as I stared at it, painful and blushing with shame. It was only a disguise, but it was on me, for life. It was there, it was there, it was real. Every one of those encounters was like a blow on the head. They left me dazed and dumb and senseless every time, until slowly and stubbornly my robust persistent illusion of well-being and of personal beauty spread all through me again, and I forgot the irrelevant reality and was all unprepared and vulnerable again.

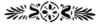

10

AT this time of secret confusion it was lucky for me that I found my brother Warren. He acted as if he did not even see my disguise. He never mentioned it, he never explained how he felt. He merely treated me as if he saw in me the growing-up proud person that I felt myself to be.

In spite of my new fierceness I was shy and in-articulate, which he was not. He was a Harvard undergraduate then, and he had just found for him-self the exhilaration and joy of intellectual exercise. He loved argument and discussion, and he loved also his own uninterrupted discourse. He could talk brilliantly and he loved to arouse and excite an admiring listener with his talk. He had the in-tellectual young man's favorite passion for influenc-ing and molding another mind, especially a young docile feminine mind, since that was the sort of mind which lent itself most willingly to be molded. He gave me such a strong impression that he was always right in his opinions that I never doubted that he was, and I felt lucky and proud to be molded and influenced by him.

He never showed off to me as he did to some of his other feminine listeners. After my father died we lived in a small countrified town outside of Salem, called Danvers, where there was almost no con-versation and no intellectual life, and the only appre-ciative audience he could find were his former high school teachers and their sisters and friends, all women. He chose this audience first because there wasn't any other, but for some reason he seemed to get some sort of very necessary nourishment and satisfaction from their uncritical worship of him. He used to love to dazzle and astonish those intelligent yet easily dazzled ladies, and he let me see that sometimes half the fun he got out of it was to start an intellectual discussion going and then laugh up his sleeve at his former teachers as they innocently fell into the trap of his arguments, and never guessed that he was amusing himself at their expense. Their

48

generous, radiant admiration of his ability was not enough. He had to make them a little ridiculous in order to enjoy himself fully. I did not understand this need of his, but I noticed how, in great contrast, he always treated me with a humility and quiet comradeship and a cherishing in which there was never anything but the utmost deference, as if he had singled me out of all the world as the only one whom he could love simply and completely. After one of the sessions of talk and argument in a spinster schoolteacher's New England salon—which might be her back porch covered with a thick green curtain of Dutchman's-pipe or her kitchen where we sat around the kitchen table and ate doughnuts—he and I would walk home together and a sudden silence would fall on us while he held my arm caressingly with his rough blunt hand. Among the women he knew, the intellectual spinsters and their admiring sisters and friends, I understood that I was his favorite. For a long time I knew that I was the only one who really mattered to him.

Yet I never could learn to talk easily with him. I do not know why it was. A fear and shyness as hard as iron barred my most important ideas and feelings out of all conversation in spite of my will and my enormous need to share them. Whenever I tried to talk I was always embarrassed, and what I said was painfully clumsy and ineffective compared with what I felt within me. Every time after we had been together I suffered unbearably from my pent-up feelings and thoughts which his companionship had excited and roused to such a pitch and which my shyness had prevented me from expressing. In order to relieve this feeling I began to write to him every

49

week as soon as he had gone back to Cambridge. For I was always at ease in writing. On paper nothing embarrassed me, nothing was too difficult or too emotional for me to try and express. But as soon as I had mailed the letter I would begin to grow hot and cold because of the things I had written. I hungered for emotional intimacy and yet when I had invited it and felt it coming toward me I was panic-stricken. I remember the real agony I felt after the first time I had written to him, whenever the postman rang, and the almost unbearable feeling when his letter actually came, and I took in my hand the heavy, fat, cream-white envelope with the crimson seal of Harvard on the flap. Opening that letter and reading it gave me a pleasure that seems strange indeed as I remember it now, because of the intensity which made it two-thirds pain. My first experience in grown-up friendship was like an awful miracle, an expansion of myself that had something of the pain of birth in it.

His letters, so cherishing, so responsive, seemed to me almost like love letters, and our meetings almost like lovers' meetings. Every Friday or Saturday he came home and, after we had begun to write to each other, he always called my name as soon as he got inside the door, as if the only thing that mattered about coming home was to know that I was there. Thus I knew then how it felt to have my company very much desired by an eager young man. And I knew the pleasure of adoring and worshiping him in return. I thought to myself very solemnly: nobody will ever love me or marry me, and so it is all right for me to feel as if this were a love affair, as it almost seems to be.

On those week-end evenings we sometimes borrowed Betty, my sister's horse, and her open buggy that had rubber tires and square kerosene lamps attached to the sides. With these dim and elegant little lights bobbing on each side of us, we drove along pitch-dark roads, out into the wide and fragrant night, out under the stars, moving slowly and, compared to the way we move now, almost imperceptibly.

Being young, we had just discovered the wonderful charm of night, night away from houses, night moving along country roads, noiseless silken wood roads, black bumpy roads of pastures and farms, and the soft, misty, sweet-smelling roads with old wooden bridges where we stopped to listen to the gentle Ipswich River. Night was a new element that we had marvelously discovered. Yet curiously it was the same element that had been only a year or two ago nothing else than a tall policeman to us, the negative tiresome dark that put an end to all our pleasures, and which my revengeful imagination had filled with insane horrors. Now we were grown up, and by the magic of transformation the great welcoming night had become our partner and our friend, the only element that was really congenial to our new selves and our new emotions.

The country round us was benign and safe for our night wanderings. It was a country of small towns and quiet villages where nobody sat up late except when there was a meeting of the local historical society or the grange. We drove past the sleeping barns and farmhouses of North Beverly and the yellow-lighted houses of Putnamville, and out onto our favorite and lonely Valley Road to Topsfield where the street lights stopped and there was nothing but the vague dark shape of trees moving slowly past us on either hand and Betty's ears bobbing up and down ahead of us, sometimes dimly visible and sometimes vanishing altogether in the darkness. With only Betty's light footsteps and the spindly wheels of our little ambling carriage to disturb the silence we were nearer to the slow clouds and the stars then in those roads than we ever have been since on any other roads. We could hear every rustle of leaves along the roadside and even the soft sound of wind in ferns. Betty carried us along with a dreamy motion and a pace that was very nourishing and kind to our mood of intimate companionship. In that dreamy silence my own stillness and shyness were no longer a handicap. We both were still, both feeling the night and listening to the night, each aware of the other's awareness and happiness as if we were two parts of the same person. Once, after such a silence, I heard my brother say, "Sometimes I wish you were not my sister."

Five or six times since I was born I have heard a sentence spoken that sounded as if it were made out of an entirely different substance from the substance of ordinary sentences, as if it were carved out of a piece of strange foreign wood. These sentences had no visible connection with what had been said before or with anything that came after them. They were undecipherable fragments, like meteorites from another world. For, as I think I have already said, I grew up in a family where a certain kind of intimate personal emotion was all so carefully hidden that it sounded to me when I heard it like a foreign language, while at the same time that it shocked and frightened me it sounded more familiar and more real than anything I had ever heard before. Those sentences were made of what George Meredith, on one crucial page of *The Amazing Marriage*, called "arterial words." They spurted out of the body involuntarily, coming from some hidden and much deeper source than ordinary speech. In our family those arterial sentences were instantly treated as if they had not been spoken. They were not answered, never repeated, and never referred to again. They were something not wanted, and something terrifyingly alive. They were foundling sentences, left on a doorstep in mid-air. We all looked the other way, we pretended we hadn't heard, and those parentless sentences were left to starve and perish, because, picked up and warmed and fed, they might have had the power to change our whole lives.

When I was young I blindly imitated the family tradition of ignoring those bursts of intimacy—I caught the contagion of our family's fear and disapproval of them. But even without the fear and the disapproval, since I was utterly inexperienced and untaught in the language of intimacy, although I felt a great hungering for the emotion and experience of it, I never in the world would have known what to do or to say in response to them.

So, when my brother said to me, after a long silence, that night when we were driving across a dark starlit place somewhere between the woods and the sea along the Beverly shore, "Sometimes I wish that you were not my sister," I recognized it for one of those strange sentences. It fell at my feet out of an unknown sky.

And I did not know how to stoop and pick it up

and hold it in my hands. This strange thing was meant for me, and for no one else, but I had absolutely no skill or grace to receive it. It was like a letter sent to a person who hadn't any name, or any street and number. I was powerless to claim it even though I knew it was mine. It set up such a commotion inside me that I could scarcely breathe.

At the first impact of it I thought he meant he hated me, and wished he never had known me. Swiftly I thought that must be because he had found at last that, although he had tried very hard, the truth was that he could not enjoy being with a deformed person, and he wished he did not have a deformed little sister to go out driving with.

"Sometimes I wish that you were not my sister." I turned it over and over in my mind, terribly wounded and dumb, and then slowly another interpretation came flooding into me. Another meaning, and if it was the true meaning these were arterial words. For if my second guess was right then what he had said to me was a very amazing thing. It was a confession that had spurted out of his body. It was not a cruel repudiation of me, but the very opposite.

Then I hastily remembered that this was something I could not let myself believe. I could secretly pretend that I had a lover in him, but I could never risk showing that I thought such a thing was possible for me, with him or any other man. Because of my repeated encounters with the mirror and my irrepressible tendency to forget what I had seen, I had begun to force myself to believe and to remember, and *especially* to remember, that I would never be chosen for what I imagined to be the supreme and most intimate of all experience. I thought of sexual love as an honor that was too great for me—not too great for my understanding and my feeling, but much too great and too beautiful for the body in which I was doomed to live. I had heard people laugh and talk about grotesquely unbeautiful women who had the absurd effrontery to imagine that men were in love with them. Even the kindest people seemed to feel that for that mistake there should be no mercy, and that such silly women deserved all the ridicule they got. In my secret meditations I pitied them because I understood, what nobody else could have guessed, how easily they could forget the cruel discrepancy between their desirous hearts and their own undesirableness. There was a curious and baffling law of nature or human nature which was very hard on them and on me. If a girl or woman was pretty her function of loving and being loved was treated seriously and sympathetically by everyone. But if she was awkward and homely and nevertheless eager for love that function seemed to be changed into something mysteriously comic and shameful. I had sworn that I never for one instant would forget the fearful discrepancy in my own case. I never would for one instant be off my guard. I never would be caught either pathetically or ridiculously imagining that anyone was or ever could be in love with me.

But I was very suspicious of my own amorousness. It was an unknown quantity in all human beings and I knew, although I had not heard of Freud then, that unknown quantity, from being forever repressed and denied, would be always waiting to trick me and betray me and make me behave without even

55

realizing it like one of those poor creatures. So now I sharply told myself that my sudden conviction that my brother meant he wished he could be in love with me was only one of those tricks of my own amorousness, and that I must have nothing to do with it.

With all this wild confusion packed inside my head I sat very still beside my brother in the little carriage. We were drawn slowly forward side by side in the starlight, all alone by ourselves in the sweet, lonely night. But after he had spoken we were as far apart as if I had been a wild animal whose distrust and fear of men even the love and good will of a kind master cannot cure.

In my sudden isolation I felt as if it were all unreal. Had he said that extraordinary thing, or had I imagined it? There was nothing in our silence to tell me. Everything seemed the same as before he had spoken. I waited, half expecting him to say a little more, so that I could be sure. But that was the end, he never said it again. He never told me what he was thinking and feeling that night, or what he thought my silence meant, that it kept him from saying any more. Perhaps he thought he had shocked me, or perhaps he decided merely that I was too immature to understand him. That foundling sentence of his died of my neglect, an atom of naked truth that was not wanted. But it never died in my mind. It never even grew misty or vague. Whenever I thought of it, even long afterward, I heard it again, as clear and startling and as incomprehensible as the first time. For it is that kind of an unanswered sentence that never does die. It stays always in our minds, ready to be remembered on the slightest provocation. It stays there always, even though it may turn into something altogether incongruous and irrelevant as our life grows and changes, a queer outlandish memento, like a piece of lava from Vesuvius lying on the parlor table.

It was a long time before that particular sentence changed into a petrified souvenir in my mind. That night when we had come in and I was alone in my room I felt a smug satisfaction because I had escaped the pitfall of making myself ridiculous or pathetic, as I was sure I would have done if I had spoken. But later on I began to be troubled by a more generous openhearted feeling. A faint, faint, persistent surmise kept coming over me that he might really have meant the grave and tragic thing that my instinct had told me he did mean. What then? Then my shameful caution and ineptitude had killed his crucial impulse to take me fully into his confidence and to tell me all about his feeling for me, whatever it was. Perhaps I had failed him in what I painfully suspected then and surely believe now is the worst way in which one person can fail another.

If I did he took it without a word or a sign, and ever afterward it was as though our usual understanding of each other had never been interrupted. Perhaps he had offered me something that was too potent and too strong for me, considering how deeply moved I was just by the ordinary tenor of our relationship. That was anything but ordinary to me. Just to be out alone with him in the night, to feel myself his unspoken favorite, was as thrilling a thing as I could bear perhaps. Our love of Nature and of the night was such a newly discovered love that it alone seemed, for me at least, to constitute a passionate intimacy between us. But whatever the real meaning of it was, that evening's episode was a turning point at which I took the wrong turn. At that moment, when my brother reached out to me and wanted perhaps to tell me the miraculous, the unbelievable thing, that I could be desired if only I would believe it—I missed the way. By my miserable silence I elected to keep on carrying the secret burden of my ignorance and despair which was to grow with time to such terrible proportions. In that moment I let my body's injury begin to infect and cripple my life.

11

IT was not strange, I imagine, that when we came home from our drives and crept upstairs to our rooms afterward I was often too excited to go to sleep. I didn't even undress and open my bed, but lay across it with my head beside the lamp and a paper and pencil in front of me. For those nights out of doors often filled me with an ecstasy that made me able to write a poem. When that ecstasy came it completely possessed me, as if my body were a musical instrument suddenly taken and played upon by an unseen hand. The boldness and strength and happiness that were natural to me and to which I was denying their natural outlet refused to be denied and to be made sickly and fearful, and they poured through my veins then in an action of delight that was healthy and bold and strong. I forgot who or where I was and I made a sort of buzzing, humming noise like a top spinning or a bee. I felt a vibration like music all through me as if my blood were actually singing. And as though I were driven by that music which was formless yet felt as if it had the force of a dynamo, I crouched over my pad and held my pencil slavishly quick and intense, ready to serve this marvelous buzzing happiness at the moment when like surcharged atmosphere it should condense and form precious words that would drop onto my paper from the end of my pencil.

I was not conscious of my buzzing until after the rapture left me. Then I heard the tail end of it, like the merry-go-round breaking down, and I thought for a split second how queer it was. But everything was queer in those days and my buzzing didn't astonish me. To me that involuntary sound was something natural, a sort of Om, the murmur of Ecstasy at the heart of things. I had found in it and my poetry a new way of worshiping the ineffable charm of life which had so troubled me and enthralled me when I was a child.

My poems were small ones, brief songs, and usually one was written complete before the rapture left me, and afterward it lay there on the paper in front of me, something visible that I could hold in my hands and admire, like a damp newborn kitten that I could lick and fondle and believe to be as wonderful as the joy in which it was conceived. It was wonderful, I thought, to have captured out of the invisible world something that was visible, a little entity, an organism, a whole thing, like a poem. Then was the only time when I felt really at ease and tranquil in the world. I used to lie and stare around me in a kind of blissful emptiness.

59

The next step in the poem's existence came the next day when, returning to my other dimension of shyness and fear, I struggled for half the day before I could bring myself to give the poem to my brother to read. He would take it into his hands very seriously as if I were honoring him with something valuable. But in spite of his deference toward me there was so much of the critic and the judge in him that I always waited in painful suspense for what he would say. Often he made some criticism, but time after time he said with quietness and authority, "That is a wonder." Once he said, "That seems to me pure genius." His praise was like a magic cloak that he put around me, canceling my predicament as swiftly and entirely as Cinderella's was canceled when she found herself dressed for the ball.

I was awed and a little frightened by his attitude toward me. He talked and talked about my writing, and from the way he talked it seemed that I had in my care something very precious for which I must be responsible. He said he thought I was a very rare person. He said I was capable of knowing and feeling great things. He said I had a destiny before me. He filled me with enormous dreams.

12

THUS the natural craving to love and to be loved turned itself into something else and found its miracle of satisfaction in my poetry and his praise, and it seemed to me that we were everything to each other. But he was a healthy vigorous young man and he needed exercise for his muscles as well as for his mind. He used to tell me about wrestling matches he took part in in Cambridge, and beer-drinking parties in Boston taverns. I listened eagerly and adoringly. It seemed to add to his distinction and importance in my eyes to know that he was living partly in a world so unknown to me. In spite of myself I was romantically curious about his new friends, those young men who reflected the masculine and convivial side of his nature, and soon he began to bring them home for week-end visits. The presence of these solemn, handsome, young strangers in our house brought me unexpected pain.

When they were introduced to me their discomfiture was as much of a shock to me as if each of them had held up a mirror for me to look at. Warren's magic cloak was snatched off me by their embarrassed glance. It showed me very plainly that there was something the matter with me, and that I was not their idea of what a friend's sister should be. If one of them happened to be left alone in the room with me for a few minutes he would hastily pick up a magazine and become painfully absorbed. While for me on the opposite side of the room those minutes seemed to expand to enormous size because of their sudden emptiness, blown up like huge, dry, empty seed pods. As my brother's favorite I felt the urgent need and desire to make an impression on his friends. I wanted to be lovely and enchanting as all sisters are in stories. I had read that when men and women are together it is the woman's part to entertain and be amusing, and if the man is shy to overcome his shyness and draw him out. My inability to play this skillful feminine role was so complete that instead of being a negative thing it was like a destructive force in Nature, it was like a dust storm or a tornado. It shriveled and exterminated any ease or charm or spontaneity which might have been in the room if I had not been there. Sometimes, however, one of the Harvard visitors would be a young man of more social experience than the others or perhaps of an inborn sympathy, and he would make an attempt to be nice to me. He would try to brighten me up with a little polite badinage, treating me as if I were a sort of interesting curiosity, a strange and intelligent child. But whether my brother's friends were embarrassed with me or kindly avuncular, I knew that when they were in the room with me they were only passing as best they could a stagnant interval until my brother should come and take them to call on the girls who lived up the street.

It was then that I first became painfully conscious of girls, when nearly every week end two or three Harvard boys came to our house. I had already begun to have longings for an intimate girl friend, and I had tentatively begun to seek acquaintance with one or two of the priggish bookish ones in our town. Now with the advent of the young men I became conscious of girls in a new and disturbing way. With my excruciatingly observant eyes I saw their long slender backs, their narrow waists, and their fascinating, mysterious little bosoms. I saw their prettiness and stylishness and the way their clothes fitted their slender womanly bodies.

I also noticed another thing, which was possessed by all girls who were what girls are expected to be. This thing was a mysterious source from which flowed an endless supply of silliness. It came in the form of lively, tireless, aimless, joking talk, about the young men, and about themselves, and about nothing. Real girls, desirable girls, I found, all were gifted with that capacity for saying whatever came into their heads and making it seem to the young men like rare entertainment. I envied everything about those lucky, delectable girls, but most of all I envied this wonderful silliness. Even though I knew it was not really amusing or witty at all by any other standard except theirs, nevertheless it was that strange silliness more than anything else which made girls correct and acceptable to the difficult and solemn young Harvard students and to that side of my brother which did not belong to me.

My brother, sauntering up the street with his friends in search of girls, had turned my new values upside down. Left at home alone now, I lay on the window seat in the room at the top of the house where he and I often spent our intimate hours, where he had discussed my poetry, where he conferred magic upon me. Now that he had deserted me the magic he had given me was not enough. Poetry became like dust in my mouth. Cruel, stupid poetry! It was only a fraud and a cheat that had deceived me into thinking that I was important, even that I was wonderful, and that nothing else mattered except poetry. Poetry was contemptible dead stuff compared with the girls who lived up the street, compared with living girls, foolish joking girls, idiotic bewitching girls. I didn't feel angry or rebellious against my brother. I accepted my lot without any question, and I went about in a state of stupid wistfulness, uncritical and uncomprehending. But I suffered consciously from a starved and desolate feeling, as a person must who is living on a diet which is very good yet which lacks one vital element that his system needs and craves. I felt starved without really understanding what I lacked. I felt starved and dumb and alone, because as usual I could not speak of my suffering to anyone.

I knew that afterward my brother would tell me scornfully how idiotic the girls were and how they bored him, and how he had only gone to see them because he had to in order to entertain his more frivolous friends. But I knew that there was something about the girls that was more important to him than he ever told me, and I would have hurled away all our sacred friendship and his great dreams for me if only I could have had instead the mysterious allure that those girls had, an allure so powerful and so mysterious that it could be utterly drenched in boring silliness and still hold my brother and his friends enslaved for hours. It was so powerful it could even transform those solemn dignified young men who were so shy with me into groveling flirtatious boys.

Sometimes I fiercely scorned and despised the girls because, having the bodies of young goddesses, as it seemed to me, their behavior was so ungoddess-like. They took for granted their physical perfection which seemed to me so unattainably and infinitely precious, and by their silliness and by their taking it so for granted they made even that perfection seem cheap and ordinary. If I had their chance, if my body had risen up, like theirs, higher each year like a young tree and blossomed finally into a miracle of completeness, dramatically prepared like theirs for

64

great experiences, what would I not have been, I thought. My mysterious anger blazed in me furiously again, in behalf of the pride and mystery of life and against what seemed to me an insult to it.

After I came to know the girls a little my brother sometimes took me with him to their houses. I used to watch and listen, sitting on one side of the room, an onlooker, never a participant in the dancing, fooling, flirting, piano playing, singing that went on. They sometimes referred to me, or asked my opinion in one of their joking arguments, and they acted toward me as if I were a mysterious little sage, a highbrow, and a very special person, never as if I were a young human being like themselves. And instead of feeling proud and scornful toward them when I was among them, I felt painfully awkward and ashamed. When they drew me into their inconsequential talk no spontaneous suitably frivolous answer ever came to my lips. I felt laborious, and heavy and unbearably solemn. But I must have sometimes said something that was funny because of its naïveté, for often they surprised me very much by laughing uproariously at some stiff shy speech of mine, which I could not see anything funny in at all. Their gaiety made me feel hideously ungay, awkward, pedantic, and utterly worthless. This feeling troubled me because it seemed to be wronging something inside me. I felt that somewhere underneath my disguise there was imprisoned a spirit even more gay and pleasure-loving than theirs.

Yet when I found that the only social success I could possibly hope for among the girls and boys of my own age consisted in my being thought cute and funny and childish, in my thirst and hunger to

65

mingle with them and to be accepted I began to cultivate in myself for these social needs the character of the appealing little clown. I slipped into the ancient role that is always expected, it seems, of the imperfect ones of the world. I was Punch, the queer little human toy, the jester at court, respected and beloved in a way in which no other kind of person is respected and beloved.

When I first began to make the boys and girls laugh by some shy burst of wit or even by an unconscious piece of naïveté I felt an outrageous glow of triumph. I was getting on. They liked me. At the same time I felt a passionate angry rebellion and shame because of my return to the childish part which I had already fiercely despised and rejected when I first felt the enormous pride and seriousness of becoming mature. If I could ever have stood up, just once, and been revealed in what I thought of as my true shape, then how my behavior would be altered! How I would show them and teach them the secret that I knew!

For I felt as if I were instinctively acquainted with a splendid style of behavior that was suitable to the beautiful perfect members of the human race, a dignity and significance in conduct and manners that these foolish boys and girls were absolutely unaware of. In my meditations that behavior reached its height between men and women in their friendship and love. What did those boys and girls know about that? I thought. I felt like a hidden burning Sappho or a Phedre who could have taught them. They might have their secret knowledge of the art of silliness that was beyond my understanding, but I felt in myself the secret knowledge or instinct that

66

makes life a wonder and a miracle. But in order to express it in myself and in my own behavior I would have to wait, I thought, until another life and another incarnation.

My feeling of despair grew much worse as Warren's acquaintance at college grew wider. I had suffered chagrin and shame in the presence of his first rather heavy girl-fancying friends. But they had no particular charm themselves with which to arouse me to a knowledge of what a strange young man's charm could be, and their interest for Warren certainly consisted only in their talent for beer-drinking and wrestling. But I learned a new and more poignant suffering when he began to bring home men like Ben Hodges, and Henry Sheahan. In these romantic figures I recognized the same quality that I felt in myself, but not hidden, not frustrated. They expressed it as naturally as they breathed, in every gesture, every tone. They were brilliant and talkative like my brother, but they were more strange and fascinating than he could ever be. They had an adventurous and wildly romantic sense of life, and a gift for building up fantastically humorous narratives out of the smallest episodes; so that they gave the impression as they sat at our dinner table and enchanted us all that their life consisted in going from one exquisitely funny experience to another. Their play with words, their effervescent mingling of sophistication with absurdity, in the manner typical of Harvard, absolutely ravished me.

These fortunate young men not only seemed to feel the excitement and charm of life themselves but they could impart it to others, with an absurd rich gurgle of laughter or an eager turn of the head. They were tall and beautiful as well, and I suffered then more than I had ever dreamed of suffering before as I fell in love first with one and then with the other. The intense pleasure that I felt while I watched and listened and adored was equaled by the bewilderment and distress of knowing that I was locked and hidden away in a prison where they could never see me or know that I was there; for I thought of myself as a responsive, gay and brilliant woman who was sitting in front of them disguised as a little oddity, deformed and ashamed and shy.

13

SO, in those first bad times, the talisman my brother gave me was not enough. He had given me intimacy of the mind, and the voluptuousness of poetry. He had tried to make it seem an honor for me to be different from the others. But I was terribly greedy, like the fisherman's wife, and I wanted more things. I did not want to be different from the others, except that I wanted all that they had and much more. Besides poetry and intimacy of the mind, I wanted the intimacy of flirtation and gaiety, the voluptuousness of dancing. I wanted to participate in life with as much freedom as they did and make out of it something more thrilling than they could ever imagine. I wanted to know everything, experience everything, I felt a continual hunger and capacity for life. I wanted somehow to get into the heart of things, whatever and wherever that might be.

Yet I remained year after year on the outside, destined, it seemed, always to watch the drama and action in other lives. And after several years of hungry onlooking, and of stupid wanderings and blind seekings, I became somehow at last (blindly and instinctively without knowing what I was doing) a very perfect imitation of a grownup person, one who was noted for a sort of peaceful wise detachment. Because of this apparently contented detachment, and a modest air of superiority, and my secret devotion to the art of writing which kept always intensifying and enlarging my world of imaginary experience, I deceived myself and everybody who knew me into thinking that I knew a great deal about life. And as my contemporaries grew matronly and burdened with family cares my curious, impersonal life seemed to give me an enviable agelessness and liberty.

And when I stumbled upon the idea that it would be a great thing for me to have a house of my own, and when I decided that the kind of a house I wanted and the only kind that would be suitable for me was a very cunning, little house, a sort of fairy-tale cottage, it must have been because the rebellious arrogant person who in youth had fought for existence inside the prison of my disguise had somehow been silenced and forgotten, had even learned to submit humbly at last, and had tried to make the most of whatever beguiling charm and appeal there might be in accepting and playing the part of a quaint, small, crumpled figure, who, something like a Walter de la Mare character, was ageless and sexless and supernaturally wise.

But the predicament had not been solved. It had merely been ignored and forgotten and left far behind me, an unopened package containing a time bomb. And now, at the composed and quiet age of just past thirty, the huge passion, the greedy enormous dream of youth which, unspent and unrecognized, had caused me such bewilderment and pain and then been somehow put aside and made unimportant, must have demanded room at last, for it knocked aside all my modest notions and took for its scene of action the high square house on an azure bay, and I unsuspectingly obeyed the order. Like someone walking in his sleep, unconsciously and dauntlessly, I think I was still looking for magic. I think I was still looking, although I didn't know it, for the secret which would transform me and restore me to my true shape.

With all my air of wisdom and knowingness I knew only one thing that was worth anything at all, I knew enough to follow a crucial instinct when it came, even though it contradicted everything that I had been or known before.

In terror and joy I went ahead with my negotiations.

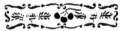

14

ON a day early in September I signed the deed, and on that great day I reached the island in my fate line and went ashore. My uneventful life began to split open, very quietly, with an invisible yet fateful movement like the opening of a seed. Sitting at a desk with a pen in my hand in Judge Patterson's office on upper Main Street where the iron deer lurks in the shrubbery, in the town of Castine, on Penobscot Bay in the State of Maine, I felt as if I had already become an entirely new person. With the signing of that document I changed from being a trifling, detached summer boarder in that town into being one of its citizens with a house and land belonging to me. That change would have been a profound one in anybody's life, but in mine it was epoch-making.

For I had become, prematurely—because I was much younger than the others, and absentmindedly because I had been walking in my sleep, inside my little shell of imitation grown-upness—one of the town's summer boarders, a race of people whose lives are finished, and who therefore are treated by the real citizens with patient compassion, as though they were not quite normal or else victims of a disaster. The abnormality or the disaster that converts normal persons at some period of their lives into chronic summer boarders, and turns them into a mild sort of nuisance and responsibility which good-hearted normal people must look after in exchange for small sums of money, consists in their apparently having no homes of their own, no occupations, and, I hate to say it but I am afraid it is true, in their being people whom nobody anywhere overwhelmingly wants or needs. They are mostly ladies, not very prosperous, not very young.

The conscious demands which these frail useless beings make on the citizens are pathetically modest, and yet just because they are the kind of beings they are, so undesired and at the same time foolishly gay and eager, their presence during two months of the summer requires great patience and forbearance on the part of normal people. When the first cold September gale comes and blows them all away, like the leaves, you can almost hear a great sigh of relief from the citizens, and a sudden feeling of tranquil, homelike sensibleness and bareness settles down all over the town.

I had been one of the worst of these parasitical creatures, because although I too was rootless and had no personal responsibilities I did not have the grace to join the others in their romantic enthusiasm for the town that harbored us during the summer. They were always running about, conspicuously gushing and exclaiming how the views there were more beautiful or the air more invigorating or the walks very much nicer than in any other town where they had previously fluttered for a season. I am sure they hoped that the stolid citizens would hear them and feel properly rewarded.

I never could say these things or feel them, simply because I didn't care for the place at all. As a summer boarder I was cold and unresponsive. I was entirely unmoved by the town's much-talked-of appeal. Somebody had put the idea into my head that its climate might do me good, and I had come and sat in its sun and air passively waiting to be done good to. And of course I got as much out of it as any scornful and indifferent person ever gets out of anything. And naturally I always felt irritated whenever I heard the sentimental ravings of my fellow boarders concerning the particular beauty and spe-

cial charm of that town. Unattached, rootless as
they were, they seemed to be still moved by a youthful, pathetic instinct for attachment. They wanted,
they tried so hard to belong there, while I did not
perceive it even for a moment as a place I would
ever take the trouble to belong to. Besides, attachment of any kind was the last thing I thought I
wanted.

Therefore the change that came over me was as
complete and sudden as a religious conversion. As
soon as I had seen my house and land and had seized
them in a powerful, willful, yet somnambulistic action, dimly yet overwhelmingly aware of what they
were going to mean to me, my own instinct for attachment suddenly awoke and possessed me and
became a furious ecstasy. I was like someone who,
having never experienced anything more than a
mild cynical flirtation, suddenly falls head over heels
in love. And the town where this miracle happened
to me became for me a miraculous town. Until then
I had never opened my eyes there, it seemed. When
I was converted I opened my eyes, and like every
convert I felt as if nobody else had ever seen what I
saw. I left every one of the special devotees far behind me in my extravagant admiration for the particular beauty and special charm of that town.

My town! I love it. The old possessive eagerness
wells up in me now as it always does whenever the
chance comes to tell about it, especially to some
person who has never heard of it before. I remember, among many other times, how this happened on
a homesick winter afternoon when I was leaning
against a cold radiator in Creteil, a Paris suburb
which lies molding in a deathly chill on the banks of

the Marne. I was talking to the young Dutch painter, Kristians Tonny, when suddenly my love for that terribly distant town welled up in me, and as I tried to describe it to him I felt such a hard, desperate need for it that he was moved just listening to me, and being from a northern country too, he seemed to understand my feeling and he acted as if there were something tragic about me, a woman in exile. Sometimes even when I was sitting absorbed in my surroundings in one of the big smoky cafés in Paris it would come over me again. Then I would have to lean forward and try to describe it to anybody who happened to be with me. Then I would think with secret sympathy of the French explorers who first discovered the site of my town on the coast of the New World. Saint Castin himself might have sat moodily in a Paris café in the continual darkness and dampness of a Paris winter after his wanderings were over, and suddenly seen in his mind's eye that brilliant coast and its luscious warm winter sun shining on snow-covered harbors and deep-blue rivers and on little purple wooded islands with rims of crumpled silver. He might have leaned forward like me in desperate homesickness and tried in vain to describe it to his companions.

I shall try again now, and probably I shall fail, as usual. The first thing about my town to me is its unique and romantic name, Castine—a name derived from the name of the discoverer Saint Castin. I cannot explain why, but the name is very important. My town could never have had the same atmosphere and the same character that it has if it were not for the sound of the name Castine. Brooksville, Winterport, Searsport, Sedgwick, Camden.

Those are the names of other villages along the same coast. I like all those names, all those towns and villages. But surely there is a difference between those names and the name Castine.

The second thing about my town is its situation. That of course was what attracted and charmed Saint Castin and all the early voyagers and discoverers, and roused in them the will to possess it. First the distinguished and intelligent tribe of Indians called the Tarratines, then the seventeenth-century seigneurs, led by Saint Castin and accompanied by Jesuit priests, and then the Dutch traders, interested in furs and fish, and then the British officers and their men, and at last the Americans—all came and fought for it one after the other and left their legend and a good many of their bones behind them.

For Castine is built on a very splendid place, worth fighting for. It is on a high, wind-swept, green peninsula barricaded with granite cliffs and washed on one side by the Penobscot River where it widens into the Bay, and on the other by a winding tidal river. Nowadays Castine is reached by land over two long roads which follow the edges of the peninsula along the shore of its two rivers. One road comes from Bucksport and Orland, keeping close to the shores of the Penobscot River, and the other skirts the salt estuary whose name is the Bagaduce, from its head in the village of Penobscot, familiarly known as the Head of the Bay. Near the wide root of the peninsula a crossroad joins the two river roads, making what is called by Castine people the Twenty-Mile Square, and farther down they are joined again by a shorter crossroad where the peninsula has grown narrower approaching its tip, and that is the Ten-Mile Square. There are no other drives in Castine. The two river roads and the two crossroads are all there are. Going either way, you pass farms sloping down to the river, deep-rooted old houses with work going on around them and geraniums in the windows; you dip up and down over wonderful round roller-coaster hills; you pass little coves circled with fields; every now and then you see a small silvery-gray deserted house with its old lilac bush and apple orchard, and crossing the Ten-Mile Square you go through a piece of woods where in spring and summer you hear whippoorwills and hermit thrushes. Driving toward Castine you have a river either way you come, and either way you come you begin to feel a wildness and excitement in the sea-surrounded air that is stirring and indescribable.

The peninsula points south, and the sun rises over one river and sets over the other. My house stood on the eastern and more sheltered side, where the sun comes up over the dark beautiful Bagaduce River and the West Brooksville hills. My house stood near the top of the slope, quite high above the river.

I used to look down and see the roofs of the fishermen's houses below me shine and steam in the morning light against the waters of the Bagaduce. Above the opposite shore I could see the delicious lilting shape of the Brooksville hills and Cape Rozier. Those rounded hills were all covered with trees, solid ranks of spruce and fir, except in one place down close to the shore where I could see against the dark background a Maine vignette in white—a little church steeple, three little white houses, and a little steamboat landing, and their still reflection in the green water below the wooden piles. The little village and its reflection across the river had the tantalizing quality of a toy scene enclosed inside a glass ball. I could almost hold it in the palm of my hand, but I could never get inside. Two or three times I went the long way round by land because I wanted so much to get there just once and to see it life-size. But through some perverse stupidity on my part I never could find the road that led down to that mysterious little church and landing, and it never once came into my mind that I could have gone over there very easily by water. I used to come back home after a long afternoon drive in search of it and stare across the water again in fond desperation. Its size was never to be altered for me, it seemed. And so again at my house, as in my bedridden childhood, I had at my side, to stare at and adore, a toy whose whole mystery and charm consisted in its wonderful littleness.

Every morning at eight o'clock and again in the afternoon a certain ancient, small, and very feminine-looking steamer, the S.S. *Goldenrod*, affectionately called the *Rod* for short, used to glide across the peaceful river to stop at the little landing and pick up a bag of mail and a passenger or two, and perhaps some article of freight. I used to like to watch the *Rod* lying against the wharf over there. She seemed to like it, and she would linger fifteen minutes or so before she glided back across the smooth bosom of the river to our old yellow steamboat landing, where she took on the rest of her passengers and mail and freight for the bold trip she made every day clear across the wide Bay to Belfast. The *Rod* was a dowdy ridiculous old lady, creaking

77

terribly in every joint, yet she always had her gloves on and her bonnet at a jaunty angle as she went careening across the Bay, bouncing ridiculously and showing her petticoats, or else primly gliding with an air of intense propriety and self-satisfaction, according to the wind.

The *Goldenrod* was not by any means the largest and most impressive ship that ever came in or out of Castine. Our harbor is very deep, so deep and spacious that a whole fleet of battleships can anchor there. But for some reason battleships and great private yachts were not, in my time, particularly interested in coming to visit us. On the Fourth of July once, I remember, a battleship came and lay in the harbor and gave us a gala celebration. And usually once or twice during every summer I used to be waked up by hearing an early morning shout of excitement ring through the house, exclaiming, "Look out the window! The *Corsair* has come in!" Then feeling a great thrill of snobbish joy I would run to the window to drink in the sight of that inhabitant of the great world of fashion and power, lying at anchor within the circle of the round Brooksville hills. But she never stayed. We had nothing to hold her, no resident multi-millionaires, no diplomatic society. At last even the Rockland steamer, the S.S. *Pemaquid,* affectionately called the *Quid* for short, gave up coming any more because her passengers grew fewer and fewer, and after that the *Rod,* and the sardine boats, and the Dennetts' motorboats taking us across to the islands on picnics and painting excursions and faithfully rescuing us in thunderstorms, and the handful of small sailboats belonging to the summer colony, were all the craft we were used to seeing in our deep, beautiful, forgotten harbor.

The village was built, of course, around the harbor, and it climbs up over the slope of the steep hill that rises above the harbor. There are Dyer's Lane, Green Street, Pleasant Street, and Main Street, four parallel streets which go up the hill. It is a long hard pull from the bottom of the hill to the top. You think you have reached the top when you come to the corner above the post office, but you are only half-way. You have to go on past the quiet and nearly empty, square, white Colonial houses and the mustard-colored and elegant Victorian houses of the aristrocracy after you cross Court Street under the elms. Past the two Miss Witherles, each alone in an ancestral house filled with a sea captain's treasures, past Mrs. Hooke and Mrs. William Walker, past Judge Patterson, whose office in the ell, near where the iron deer stands, is a sunny room where the smell of old law books and of a hot Franklin stove made a rich, exciting atmosphere on the crisp fall morning when I signed my deed; past Miss Lucy Grey, a lonely and refined old graduate of Wellesley, past Dr. Babcock, past Dr. Philbrook, the homeopathic doctor, who made wonderful fish-chowder suppers for his friends; and finally at the top of the hill past the house of my friend Captain Patterson, who at eighty climbed that long hill with ease twice a day, coming home to dinner and to supper all the way up from Dennett's Wharf. Here at Captain Patterson's house Main Street ends and the golf links begin, where the summer colony's Victorian clubhouse stands. Here you have come to the High Road, which runs along the topmost ridge and backbone

79

of the peninsula, and here the cold, sea-smelling wind slams against you from across the links and from across the wide stretch of water that lies between Castine and Belfast. It is a town of extremes. On summer days the bottom of Main Street is often hot and sultry while at the top there is ice in the air.

On the edge of the links you will see a series of grassy windswept mounds with a flat top and square corners, like very large graves. Those green mounds are all that is left of Fort George, built by the British when they took the peninsula during the Revolution. The boys of the present generation still know how to crawl down into the dungeon under the fort where the American drummer boy was held a prisoner all alone and kept on drumming as long as the life was in him. The drummer boy was only fourteen years old, they say, and he drummed for three days and nights until he died of hunger and thirst and exhaustion, or as some say until he was killed and eaten by enormous rats. Every year in the last week of August when the moon is full, as it was at the time he perished, you can hear him drumming again for three nights underground. By the middle of August the people of Castine begin to mention him in their conversation. "It's almost time for the drummer boy," they say, as if they were saying "It's almost time for the corn to be ripe." Intellectual ladies in the summer colony discuss him from a scholarly point of view and compare notes on who has heard him other years and exactly where and at what hour. My tall, pretty cousin Miriam heard him one summer about fifteen years ago when she was sitting in the moonlight at an evening picnic beside Moore's Rock. She has believed in him ever since.

And I remember one night when I was staying at
the Brophy Cottage boardinghouse Mary Goodwin
flew in there breathless and wide-eyed. She had run
all the way through a short cut from the High Road
between some alder bushes, hearing the drummer
boy just over her shoulder with every step she took.
And my niece Harriet still remembers at twenty just
how the drummer boy sounds because she heard
him when she was only four. Her nursemaid, a
Castine girl, took her on one of those three haunted
August afternoons to sit by the fort on purpose to
hear him, and Harriet after sixteen years declares
with sober conviction that she heard him. A serious
pitying look comes into her face as she tells me how
weird and frightening that sound was. I suppose
there is no other sound that could be mistaken for a
drumbeat under the earth. I wish that I could say
that I have heard it too, but I believe in it because
of the way Harriet looks when she remembers it,
and because of the way Mary looked when she burst
into the Brophy Cottage parlor.

The townspeople, the native citizens, believe in
him of course, but he is an old story to them, and I
don't think they often think about him except at the
brief time in their lives when they are young and
flighty. Then the interest which some of them take
in him is not exactly academic. On those three
moonlight nights a handful of the craziest boys and
girls of the town make him an excuse to sit up all
night on the fort. They amuse themselves by daring
each other to go down into the dungeon, and they
roam over the links together laughing and talking
in the bright moonlight, and every few yards one of
them will suddenly stop and jerk all the others back.

81

They stand still and listen and make believe they hear him. Sometimes in the midst of their irreverent horseplay one of them does hear him. Then the girls scream and laugh hysterically and start to run away from the deep shadow of the moonlit fort, and the boys catch them and won't let them go. It is rather a wild game, in which their fear of the supernatural and their rowdy amorousness play upon each other and heighten each other as the moonlit night hours pass, and sometimes a child is born the following spring to very young and irresponsible parents who could claim the drummer boy as a sort of godfather.

Beyond Fort George and the links are the Witherle Woods, and beyond the woods are the cliffs, eighty feet high. When you come out of the woods and out onto the top of the cliffs it is like the sudden opening of a door. The wind hits you and stiffens against you with its full force and you stand and stare and marvel at the expanse of blue. It is here on the western side of the peninsula that the great Penobscot River joins the Bay, winding spaciously between high wooded shores. It is on this wind-beaten tip of the peninsula, called Dyce's Head, where a little whitewashed lighthouse rises into the sunlight out of dark fir trees and the clang of the bell buoy is always and forever in your ears, that the summer people have their cottages. Their shingled roofs are soaked in fog and spray, and their glass-enclosed porches are pounded by an enormous wind that is almost never still. The wind gives its character to Dyce's Head on its days of absence nearly as much as by its almost continual presence. When it veers around or drops entirely you feel what seems like a supernatural quietness taking its place.

I remember how on those rare windless days I used to lie in a grassy hollow on top of the cliffs in front of the Goodwins' cottage and soak myself in the sun, and smell the sweetness that the hot, still air brings out of the surrounding fir balsam trees. On those days the waves used to move very gently against the rocks at the bottom of the cliffs, and the bell buoy gave a slow drowsy clang, not wild and hysterical as on other days. Lying on top of the Goodwins' cliffs was like lying on a shelf hung between the sea and the sky.

This was all I knew of Castine in the beginning— the cliffs, and the Brophy Cottage boardinghouse, and an occasional drive around the Ten-Mile Square. I was a passive and unawakened and vir- ginal summer boarder with no attachment to any- thing. My eyes had never yet dwelt with faithful tenderness upon the little village on the opposite shore of the Bagaduce, and my mind had never yet imagined any such devotion to that place as was later to enrich my life. But even in my period of black ignorance I knew enough to adore the Good- wins' cliffs. Sometimes at night, the time when it is most frightening and most wonderful to lie there in the darkness between the sea and the sky, I think I began to be dimly aware of the genius loci which inhabits Castine.

This genius loci is linked with the drummer boy, but it is much more general and all-pervasive than he is—it is a wonderful and mysterious something in the air of Castine. It is always there, but every year toward the height and fullness of summer, at the time of the drummer boy, this something seems to reach its height and fullness too. It comes at the time of year when driving at night you pass those rustling dark jungles of ripe corn which in late August seem to have sprung up overnight in the fields along the Ten-Mile Square, and when the Aurora Borealis begins to appear, like a ghostly army waving spears all over the north sky. This genius loci is a strong unseen presence, which if we were ancient Greeks would surely be given the name of a god and be honored by us with an altar in the Witherle Woods; because it is an influence which takes quite simple, everyday human beings out of themselves and astonishes them during that short, exciting season, with the sudden acquisition of many charming personal qualities they never had before. In those last sultry days and nights in August, every year, the Witherle Woods, the Goodwins' cliffs, the shores and the fields of the Ten-Mile Square, and some of the nearer islands of Castine, are filled by a powerful invisible something which makes that peninsula more alive and more stimulating than ordinary places are. The result is a kind of intoxication among the people who happen to be there. The native-born, like the crazy boys and girls who roam the links to listen to the drummer boy, yield to it instinctively without any great change in their habits; but it is interesting to see how under its influence the behavior of hitherto conventional, cautious summer visitors can be completely disrupted and can give way to a mood of unprecedented personal allurement and joyous abandon, which they generally lose again after those two or three weeks are over. It is lovely to see in otherwise brittle and conventional people and their lives this short interval of boldness and gaiety and this incandescent glow as if some ancient primitive aphrodisiac charm were working on them. In fact, it is difficult, seeing such things happen there which never could have happened in any ordinary place, not to be struck with the idea that one of the very old pagan spirits must still cling to this place, as faithful as the drummer boy and more ancient, left over since long before the French and the Jesuit fathers came, when the Indians and their gods had it all to themselves.

When I first came there I didn't know about the havoc that the genius loci of Castine was capable of causing. I only knew that the real summer people who owned houses there and had come year after year for many years seemed to feel and understand something more concerning their favorite town than could actually be seen. There was some kind of a hidden fascination about it which the real initiates were aware of as nobody else was. And it was a secret thing. They couldn't speak of it, or even try to explain it to anyone else who hadn't consciously felt it too. It was uncommunicable. The poor unattached summer boarders innocently fluttered and gushed in their devotion to it, but more than that of its potent action they never could have guessed or dreamed of. All that I myself knew in the beginning was that in the woods around the Goodwins' house and in the wind that blew around their cliffs there was something specially exciting and wonderful.

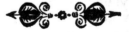

15

IT was because of Mary Goodwin, and her devotion to the cliffs and the solitude and the stillness and the wind, that in the beginning I knew the tip of the peninsula more intimately than any other part. Mary had spent all the nineteen summers of her life there in her mother's cottage next to the lighthouse, and she used to tell me about it during a winter that I spent in bed in a Boston hotel apartment. That winter, for an unknown reason, my heart was beating much faster than was good for it, rest had been ordered, and I was being kept in bed month after month. Nobody ventured and I least of all would have ventured to try to uncover the unacknowledged thing which only my heart knew about and to which only my heart was giving the needed expression, with no help or sympathy from my mind. For a long time I had kept myself coolly detached from any feelings of sorrow or frustration, and I was beginning to crystallize into a cheerful spinsterhood. Therefore I didn't listen to what my heart was trying to tell me about myself. I wouldn't listen when destiny sent Mary to me to guide me in the right direction, just as God once sent the great whale to guide and enlighten one of His most inattentive and disobedient children.

In the beginning of our friendship I felt surprised that anyone so young as Mary should like me, for she was only nineteen and I was twenty-nine. Her youth made me suddenly feel uncomfortable and unsure of myself. For I had always avoided meeting beautiful and worldly-looking girls with the same

care and intensity with which I had invariably noticed and stared at them from a safe distance. In
theaters and restaurants I always picked them out
from among the ordinary people and lost myself in
contemplation of them, almost as if I left my own
body and entered into theirs. The ones who looked as
if they were good or intellectual did not interest me.
I liked to watch only those who looked as if they
were bad, that is, sensual, cruel, and worldly. I
liked the ones whose arrogance gave them absolute
ease and simplicity of movement. I would watch a
ravishing beauty go slowly down the aisle of a theater, with her evening cloak hanging off her shoulders and her escort hovering close behind her. I
would watch her turn and go into the row where
their seats were, and as she moved with cool non-
chalance toward her place I could see for a moment
her profile or her full face. I would stare at her even
after she sat down, when all I could see was her
hair, her neck, and her shoulders, and the profile
of her escort's face turned toward her smiling, while
she coldly disregarded him for a moment until she
chose to turn and reward him. It was her purity of
movement as she came in that I deeply admired,
and then after she sat down, her essence of stillness
—nothing unsure, nothing faltering. In contrast with
that perfection I looked with contempt upon the
way the rest of the audience took their seats—I hated
the fussy, broken, clumsy movements of elderly
ladies or of vulgar young ones, as they went bobbing
or prancing down the aisles, and then, once seated,
their perpetual twisting and turning and fluttering
of hands, and heads, and shoulders. My eyes would
go back from them to the absolute calm and stillness

of my beauty. In public places, for I never met them in my private life, wherever one or more of these exalted beings were to be seen, I always picked out one among them and identified myself with her. For in such a girl I remembered something which I had forgotten until each time when I saw her again. I remembered the person whom I secretly, childishly believed I had been meant to be. As I stared at her I felt toward that regal girl a prescience, a clairvoyant intimacy, as if I had been she in another incarnation. In part of myself, I believed, *I knew*, that either I had once been able or without my present fatal disguise I would now be able to feel and look and move the way she looked and moved, as destructively and cruelly perfect and calm and exalted as she, who by her entrance made the rest of the audience suddenly change into a crowd of shapeless, comic, wriggling caricatures of human beings. In order to stir me deeply and to give me the illusion of my affinity with her, my interchangeableness with her, it was necessary that she should not show any signs of possessing any of the things which were valued in my world, such as a bright mind or a sense of humor. It was necessary for my admiration that her miraculously perfect physical flowering should be combined with superb coldness and arrogance. The possession of sheer beauty and its powerful action on others must be her only gift. Whenever I occupied a seat in a theater I had to slyly manage to sit on one of my own feet in order to lift me up a little higher, and also I had to stuff a part of my coat under me, furiously intending that nobody should notice my tricks. Without them I could not see over the top of the seat in front of me, much less over the other people's shoulders and around the backs of their heads. Even with these awkward and clumsy devices of mine, my foot and ankle aching painfully after an hour or two in that position, I was not any higher than a ten-year-old child; and yet from this humiliating level I utterly forgot the little locksmith that I was, while my eyes, just clearing the tops of the seats in front of me, made me believe that in the conspicuously beautiful and regal girl I was gazing at, who was in everything the very antithesis of me, I was staring at my own defrauded self and feeling vicariously my own rightful feelings of proud separateness and ease in contrast to the crowd of fidgeting, homely people around us.

Because of this memory or this illusion of identity, nothing would have induced me to face one of these fortunate contemporaries of mine. I owned a little arrogant set of substitutes for those things which I believed were really mine, and these sustained my self-esteem in the world I lived in, which after all was not even that world of fashion where I felt that my other self belonged. In the world I lived in my talents and my jokes and my mask of childish charm were always treated as evidence that I was a superior and valuable human being. In order to maintain my own beguiling jolly feeling of superiority I could not afford to let anything shatter my precious little set of substitutes. I had to stay always carefully among the kind of people, the literary and artistic people, or the humble, simple people, who valued my various exhibits. Most people I ever met did seem to value them, and my self-esteem rarely suffered. There were in fact only two kinds of persons, and they were really one kind, who could destroy me and all my little tricks with one casual glance. They were that heartless and worldly and beautiful young woman, wherever I saw her, whoever she happened to be, and the adoring young man who inevitably accompanied her. As long as they were unaware of me I could stare at them and forget myself utterly as I merged in them, but I could never let it happen that they should look at me or speak to me. For I knew from experience that if they should merely pass by me near enough for either of them to give me an accidental, instant's glance, that glance, first of cold curiosity and then of immediate dismissal, would tell me as cruelly and explicitly as words could have done that by their ruthless standard I didn't even exist. Whenever that glance touched me I could not deceive myself; I knew as they knew that my substitutes were worthless, that as a young, feminine human being I was a grotesque, pitiable failure, and there was no help for it. One such encounter destroyed all my defenses as one bomb destroys a building, but they were no sooner all in ruins around me than I began to repair and build them up again with a curious, indestructible persistence. But it was much pleasanter not to have the bomb hit me.

Although Mary Goodwin was young, and beautiful, and worldly-looking, yet she never gave me that destroying glance, for there was something lovably obtuse about her. She didn't seem to notice my age, my old maidism, or even my physical imperfections. I soon discovered that she herself was shy and rebellious and ill at ease in the rich, correct, Episcopalian world she was born in. It was not an intellectual rebelliousness, but the rebelliousness of a hu-

morous but uneasy child who does not understand
his own uneasiness; and she expressed it like a child
by willfully annoying and shocking the conventional
people around her. She expressed anger and jealousy
and love with childish violence and simplicity which
made her unpopular with her contemporaries. She
was erratic and reckless and innocent, she existed
in a dream, and she had soft, excited eyes.

I was fascinated by her continual devotion to her
face. She was the first person I had ever known of
the generation which was responsible for introduc-
ing the art of make-up into good social standing. It
was an entirely new thing in those days, such deliberate painting and powdering. It seemed very dangerous, as if it must surely lead to immoral adventures, and was therefore very fascinating for me, an
uninitiated spinster, to watch. She was always having to go to the nearest mirror to put on fresh mas-
cara. She beat her powder puff over her face with
such violence and lavishness that the front of her
black dress was always dusty with it. Besides being
untidy and irresponsible, she was absent-minded and
forgetful and always late. These shortcomings and
her complete innocent unawareness of them struck
me when they came into my spinsterish, orderly life
as being refreshingly novel things. This probably
explains why she was not uneasy with me and liked
me. I was the first grown-up person who never tried
to change her. I was amused and fascinated by her
exactly as she was. Sometimes she had the odd
charm for me of making me feel young and ignorant.

When she had finished her maquillage and was
brushed off and ready to go out she was to me almost
terrifyingly beautiful. She was beautiful because of

the way her face was made and because of the eyes she had, and she was worldly-looking because of her determined, serious efforts to be so. She wore black, Parisian clothes and a small string of pearls, and she almost succeeded in her ambition to look at nineteen like an experienced woman, but was hindered by her naïve self-consciousness and shyness. These stood in her way very badly with the men she really liked and wished to conquer. She had her bold, amazing flirtations with enthusiastic taxi drivers and admiring maîtres d'hôtels, but in her own world she was paralyzed with shyness and could not speak. Therefore, of course, I could never really be afraid of her, even in her most beautiful and successful moments. Also she had an endearing way of remembering me and noticing me even when she seemed most absent-minded and unobservant. She always treated me as if I were something rare and valuable in her eyes. She would interrupt one of her long silences by suddenly exclaiming, "I adore you, Kitty!"

Of all I liked about her the thing I liked the most was her laugh. It was a scarcely noticeable laugh at first. It consisted of a sudden, responsive shine in her eyes and a soft, murmurous giggle in the same tone as her speaking voice, which was of the husky, torch-singing kind. She talked very little, and she expressed most of her feelings of appreciation or sympathy or pleasure by that laugh and a childish jerky nod of the head. I must have done most of the talking because the two things I remember more than anything else about the times when she used to come and sit with me are her silence and the monotone of her laugh making an accompaniment to whatever I was telling her. Her laugh was one of the

nicest sounds I had ever heard, and belonged to the
category of certain primevally sweet and strangely
touching sounds whose charm you cannot ever really
account for. It belonged to the same family of sounds
as the murmuring of pigeons that I used to hear on
the hotel window sill that spring.

One reason why she talked so little was because
she was afraid of me, she told me afterward. I impressed her at first as being terribly sophisticated
about writing and writers, which awed her and attracted her too, because next to having romantic
adventures she wanted to be a Bohemian and a
writer. But she would always begin to talk without
shyness whenever she happened to think about
Castine. I am sure I must have thought then that she
was quite as expressive about Castine as anyone
needed to be. This was only because I never got
from anything she told me any vision of Castine or
the faintest foreknowledge of what Castine was
going to do to me. But now as I look back I can see
that she was describing that maddening place with
the same inarticulate and helpless love with which
years later I stumblingly and frantically tried to describe it myself to strange people in strange places.

That long winter in bed in Boston was made forever memorable for me by two things Mary did. She
brought me a pair of foolish, beautiful lovebirds
whom we named Ethel Monticue and Mr. Salteena,
or the Young Visiters. The minute domestic and
amorous life of these two young "visiters" in their
red cage I found as entertaining as a long domestic
novel by Arnold Bennett. It helped me to pass the
time just as an endless novel would have done.
Second, she obstinately insisted that I should go to

Castine. In May, when it began to be hot in the city, her mother came up from Hartford to see her and called on me with Mary and brought me an official invitation to Castine. I decided that I was not quite well enough to be a guest, but before the summer was over I had made the journey, with Ethel Monticue and Alfred Salteena, and installed myself in the Brophy boardinghouse.

I stayed for two consecutive summers, and the best part of those summers Mary and I spent together on her cliffs, with the wind and the sound of the bell buoy in our ears. Mary wrote poetry and read it aloud to me, and I dreamed about the endless novel I was writing. Mary was always hopelessly, speechlessly in love with somebody, and we would talk for hours on the cliff about her adored one, who somehow never quite noticed her or, what was almost worse, noticed her only until he noticed someone else more. But we both knew that something wonderful would happen to Mary. She was much too beautiful and loving for it not to happen. She felt the same greedy longing for experience and the same convictions about her capacity for love as I had once felt about myself; but hers were legitimate desires and convictions, I thought, while mine, it seemed, were not legitimate because of my deformity, and I had renounced them. Because of my years I felt older and wiser than Mary, but in actual experience I was as ignorant and young as she. The cliff proved to be a point of departure for both of us. Like two chrysalises, passive and still and waiting, we sat on the cliff rapt in the dreamlike, trancelike unreality which is the prelude to experience for every imaginative being. After that perfect prelude the moment for action came to Mary and me simultaneously at the end of the second summer, in the season of the drummer boy. Then we both took the dramatic leap into our lives and our futures. Mary went with me to Judge Patterson's office on the September day when I signed the deed to my house and land, and then she left for Hartford to marry Willy and sail for Paris.

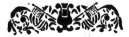

16

THERE was something about the way the Goodwins lived there in their house on the cliff which I enjoyed at first without being aware of its source. It came from Mrs. Goodwin, who had a fundamental need or gift for etiquette, which made it not merely something superficial but a means of delicate, personal expression like one of the arts. By using her need or gift she put fresh meaning and unexpected charm into everyday actions and in doing so enhanced and preserved for other people, as painters and writers do, certain places or incidents which otherwise would have passed by unnoticed. In her hands the routine of daily life seemed like a fine material that she was weaving. She was as faithful and unobtrusive as a good craftsman, keeping her hand and her watchful eye always upon her household, so that it never lost for a moment its smooth and accurate style or its quality of romantic nostalgia. Even a newcomer like myself felt the romantic nostalgia in all the ceremony of their summer life on the cliffs.

When they first came there the Goodwins' love of the place had expressed itself in certain spontaneous, happy adventures which later grew into a ritual, which became increasingly important with the passage of time, because, by linking each new summer with all that were gone, it brought the past, happy years back again. It was evident that this ritual which she kept alive by her creative touch and her constancy preserved the happiness of earlier summers spent with her little children who were now grown and with their father whom they and she adored and who had died in the midst of life. The children were as constant as their mother and had never grown away from the Castine past, for they all felt that something precious would be lost if any of their ritual were changed, or left out, or forgotten, or neglected.

This united constancy made me remember that my own life lacked something essential, for we had once had a family ritual in Stowe. But we had lost it. We had sold the little Bigelow farm and nothing had ever taken its place in our lives again, and I felt an orphanlike thrill when I found myself adopted by the Goodwins and taking part in their family ceremony. It didn't matter at all that I was a newcomer. It was taken for granted and correctly that the importance of the family customs and ceremonies and sentiments would be immediately apparent to me and excite my instant desire to participate and belong. Mrs. Goodwin never neglected a young newcomer in her house, as preoccupied parents often do, but took pains to have intimate talks with

me as if she wanted to establish independently of
Mary a friendship between us. In a little ceremony
of introduction she took me out on the top of the
cliffs when I first came; and by telling me a few little
things about the past summers and by a sudden
slight, involuntary coming of tears into her eyes as
she spoke she gave me a deep perception, almost
without any words at all, of what her marriage and
her children and her husband meant. She seemed to
feel that as her guest I had not been entirely admitted and could not share and fully enjoy the wonderful quality of the place until she had given me a
glimpse of her personal history of happiness and
love. With flattering, simple candor she did this for
me, shy and isolated and hungry for intimacy as I
always was.

I loved all the family picnics at the long-estab-
lished favorite places, the motorboat lunch picnics
at High Head or at Indian Bar, the swimming tea
picnics at Craig's Pond, the painting picnics on the
hill in Penobscot, and the all-day excursions, sometimes by automobile to Bangor or Bar Harbor, and
at other times on board the S.S. *Goldenrod* to Belfast
across the Bay. But the best and most characteristic
of all the institutions were the evening suppers on the
rocks at the foot of the cliffs. The guests and the family and the smiling maids, who were always skillfully
initiated into the ritual, went in single file down the
long wooden staircase against the face of the cliff in
rosy sunset light, carrying the baskets of food and
the special outdoor frying pans and the lumberman's
coffeepot and the hot biscuits made in the house and
wrapped up in warm napkins. The great flat rocks
we picnicked on were only a few inches above the

97

deep surge of the Bay. As darkness came over us it was frightening and beautiful to be sitting on that ledge, almost on a level with deep water, the cliffs rising up high over our heads, and far across the darkening Bay the black coast line, where soon the lights of Searsport and Belfast began to twinkle. The perilous wildness was made more thrilling by the safety and coziness which Mrs. Goodwin cast around us like a magic shawl. If we had been shipwrecked on a desert island I felt sure she would have been able to produce a perfectly equipped and generously packed tea basket; and punctually at four o'clock she would take out her canister of tea and a box of waterproof matches and would light the spirit lamp; and while she was waiting for the kettle to boil she would further astonish us by producing a traveling pillow of exactly the right shape and size to put at our backs. She would begin to talk to us soothingly and when we were ready for it ask sympathetic questions about ourselves and our lives until presently the fact that we were shipwrecked on a desert island would have entirely escaped our attention.

She made life a downy nest in which her family and guests could recline and lose whatever small sense of responsibility we might otherwise have felt. During those luxurious summers absent-minded Mary and my passive, enchanted self used to take possession of the top of the cliffs and lie in the sun and listen to the bell buoy and read and write and talk to each other and forget the hour until Mrs. Goodwin sent a maid out to tell us it was time for lunch or tea. Or else she sent a tray to us, which she herself probably had set, for it was done with care and imagination and the food was of a kind to satisfy a poet's gusto for nourishment and also his notoriously difficult standard of perfection. We were humored and spoiled, and I thought it was very fine indeed, for the careless, absent-minded young to be sheltered during their season of absent-mindedness in such a careful chrysalis. For in too many houses the life of the mind, when it is just beginning to discover its individual existence in the young members of a family, often has to accommodate itself to the unnecessary, senseless tyranny of the domestic machinery, as if it only were the all-important thing. And in such a household any young person who instinctively tries to shelter his mind's life with a little private margin of stillness and solitude and timelessness is likely to awaken a curious resentment and even hatred in more practical members of the household, as though they were jealous of the prestige and latitude sometimes accorded to those who indulge in meditation.

In other houses that I had known where the life of the mind was considered of first importance the life of the body was taken care of in a very haphazard fashion. When I first lived among artists and writers I learned to my surprise that those notoriously impractical people were able to produce meals far better than any I had ever tasted. I was awed by their epicurean knowledge and skill, and I was delighted also by the long irregular periods between these superb meals when everything was helter-skelter and there were no real meals at all. I adored their easygoing disregard of rules which I had always found so irksome and distasteful, but which I had supposed were unavoidable. Their revolutionary and to me highly congenial sense of what was important thrilled me. Absorbing discussions about painting and writing, or the mood for working, were considered too important to be interrupted by any arbitrary schedule of eating and sleeping. But I soon found to my dismay that I did not have the physical reserves necessary to live in such style. After a day or two of haphazard meals and insufficient sleep my body drooped and wilted like a neglected child's. The illness which had forced obedience and patience on me for so many years had made me hate restraint and hate the sensible, stupid people who were always trying to impose it. But that illness—although past now—had damaged my body too severely ever to bear any unusual physical strain. So after one or two experiments I had to surrender again to the dull prosaic life of regular and careful habits, but in my heart I was even more rebellious.

My antagonism against sensible people went much deeper than mere rebellion against any sort of restraint. I did not like the way they placidly took it for granted that physical comfort and health and financial security were the only really important things in the world, and were ignorant of the beliefs and passions of the head which may require a person to abandon security and health and comfort and sacrifice his reputation or even his life if necessary. I longed fiercely to prove my contempt for safety when it was considered of greater importance than spiritual and intellectual freedom. I did not want safety for its own sake, but only in order that I might keep my body alive and my mind clear long enough to say or do what was in me to say or do.

In Mrs. Goodwin's house I discovered that hunger

and fatigue and the need for physical order could be satisfied by a housekeeping which was like a work of art, as accurate and formal and pretty as a ballet, but which still left the mind with all the scope it wanted, to be both free and sheltered at the same time. I knew that when I got a house of my own I would wish to create in it a climate equally congenial to the mind which would possess something of the perfection Mrs. Goodwin had achieved.

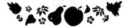

17

I SIGNED the deed just as the summer season ended and my boardinghouse was about to close. I went immediately to call on my new unknown neighbor. I told her I had just bought the house next door to hers, and I asked her if she could let me have a room in her house for a few weeks while I was having repairs and changes made. After a little gentle nervousness and hesitation she consented and said she thought her married daughter, Lorna Clement, who lived across the road would be willing to give me meals.

I looked with eager and interested eyes upon my new neighbors, Mr. and Mrs. Douglas. I would have liked them whatever they had been, because they were the first neighbors of my own that I had ever had. They were not my family's neighbors, but my own, Katharine's, just as the house was my own personal enterprise. In the ardor and novelty and freshness of my joy I felt that our relationship would be something unlike what anybody else had ever achieved toward neighbors. I had an enormous faith in my own way of doing everything, now that I had begun at last. I had an idea that I could make something rare and wonderful out of whatever material I was to find. And I knew the moment I saw the Douglases that I had been lucky in the material.

Mr. Douglas had bright-blue eyes and a ringing, welcoming, cordial voice, which pealed forth in song from the Unitarian church choir every Sunday morning. He had an elegance and style of manner which for some reason usually seems incongruous in a countryman. But it was not a city elegance. He called Mrs. Douglas "Wife" when he spoke to her, just like a woodcutter in a Grimm's fairy tale, who lives in a cottage on the edge of a forest. Most conveniently for me, however, Mr. Douglas was a farmer who sold milk and vegetables. Mrs. Douglas welcomed me with an affectionate look which was also a little vague and absent-minded. She was one of those rare, slender, middle-aged ladies in whose face and way of moving and talking you can see more clearly the very feminine young girl of the past than you can see the fifty- or sixty-year-old woman who is supposed to have taken her place. She had not acquired the thick disfiguring shell within which most of the boys and girls of a generation ago are so cleverly concealed that you can hardly believe they ever existed. With Mrs. Douglas the shell was so thin that you could look right through it and see, only slightly blurred, the soft, innocently engaging absent-minded girl. I felt drawn to her as if she had been an unprotected wistful person, although she had the protection of a devoted family and certainly did not need me. But I felt that nobody, not her family and surely not me nor any stranger, could ever get close to her, because the thing in her which made her seem young and in need of protection also made her seem far away and inaccessible. Lorna told me afterward that her mother had lost a child, her youngest, and had never recovered from the loss. When I learned that, I knew it must be the reason why she seemed the way she did. She had refused to leave the period in her life when she still had the little boy, I thought. She had stayed behind with him and therefore remained essentially young and unchanged herself, while all the rest of the family had gone on into the future and grown older.

When she and Mr. Douglas talked to me, discussing my house, and I told them my plans and asked them to tell me about carpenters and painters they knew, I was delighted to hear in their voices the inflection which I had learned to recognize as one of the unique characteristics of Castine. Their voices kept going up and down, up and down, indulgent, humorous, and persuasive, no matter what the subject of the conversation might be. The effect of this inflection is that even in the most casual remark the inhabitants of Castine always seem to be insisting gently and humorously that they want to comfort you for everything and want to excuse you for all your faults. "There, there, everything is all right, don't you be frightened or upset about anything," say the men's voices, as well as the women's voices, no matter what they are saying. I was crazy about that sound. It was just what I had been needing all my life to hear. I think of it as one of the physical elements of Castine, like the Castine air, which the inhabitants are so used to breathing that if they have to go away they discover to their surprise that they cannot breathe well in other places. In the same way they become so spoiled by the sound of reassurance in every local voice that when they go to cities they are painfully surprised by what seems like inhuman harshness or at best a very strange indifference toward them in their casual encounters with people. Even swearing sounds benevolent and loving in Castine. The men seem to put an almost feminine note of humorous, indulgent caressing into their curses, which are certainly richer and more abundant in their talk than any I ever heard before. This interesting characteristic, I thought, could only be found among people who know human nature intimately and have decided to laugh and excuse it all. I soon learned to use the accent myself in an amateur fashion and without the background of experience it implied.

On the morning when I came over to stay at Mrs. Douglas's house, bringing all my things with me from the boardinghouse, she got me settled in my room and then she took me across the road to her daughter's to introduce me. We had reached Lorna's porch steps when Lorna came out of her door. She was ardent and young-looking in her early thirties. Taller than I, of course, and two or three steps above me, she leaned over to shake hands and she spoke to me in a merry excited voice that sounded like a blackbird or a robin, it was so rich and round. As she leaned over me I was aware of a sudden strong rush of feeling coming from her toward me, of compassion and sweetness. I felt that she gave me her loyal friendship then and there, wholly and without any hesitation. This amazed me, especially the compassion. As I have said already, I had a chronic sense of my own well-being and good fortune. It never occurred to me, except when I was forcibly reminded of it by something outside myself, that there was anything about me which could make anyone feel sorry for me. On that day especially I felt so lucky, so rich and enviable, that I could only regard objectively her strange compassionate warmth toward me, deciding that she possessed the kind of heart which needs to embrace and pity the whole world.

Besides, my attention was quickly all taken up with her, not myself. I knew the minute I looked at her that she was wonderful. I thought she had one of the loveliest faces I had ever seen. I told her I liked her short hair, which only rather sophisticated women had begun to wear then. She laughed with great amusement at my liking it and told me she had cut it herself that very morning because her husband wanted her to. She added vehemently that she thought it looked awful and she was dreadfully ashamed of it. I couldn't take my eyes away from her. I was delighted with the distinguished look the straight cut gave to her already distinguished face. I noted with pleasure and pride that my neighbors the Douglases and Clements all had beautifully modeled faces. Lorna's face might have belonged to a member of some cultivated aristocratic family in the best period of its intellectual and spiritual flowering. Her housedress and apron and her plain unassuming air filled me with wonder at the contrasts to be met with in the world.

As soon as her mother left us Lorna and I immediately began to tell each other all about ourselves like two schoolgirls. We began then the endless conversation which went on for weeks and months and years. I sat down on the woodbox in the kitchen so as to be near her and talk to her while she was moving around doing her work. My choice of the woodbox instead of the nice little rocking chair she offered struck her as being very droll and amusing. She laughed again just as she had laughed when I admired her haircut. Whenever I had a chance to perch on something higher than an ordinary chair I always did, instinctively, without thinking about what I was doing. For when I sat on an ordinary chair it reduced my face and eyes to a level much lower than that of the normal person sitting in a chair. This situation is curiously outraging to the normal sense of physical self-esteem—it gives a grown-up person a childish and inadequate feeling which I had always felt obliged to cancel by making a laborious display of a gay triumphant personality. It is much easier to sit on something higher and feel adult and debonair without so much effort. It happened that Lorna's woodbox was just the kind of seat I liked and could feel gay on. In the happy confiding mood in which our friendship began, something about the enthusiastic manner in which I took possession of the woodbox and told Lorna that I liked it much better than a chair, without bothering to explain to her the reason or even to think about it, seemed to her delightfully capricious and amusing; and from that day on she always indulgently offered me the woodbox and I always sat on it while we talked in her kitchen. When she had finished her work we used to go into her little sitting room and sit in front of the Franklin stove, while we went on with our never-ending speculations about life and told each other old wives' tales about people we had known.

In the beginning our point of departure was the subject of my house. I had begun to interview carpenters and painters, and I was curious to know something about the different ones I met. Lorna always had some strange, funny, or pitiful thing to tell me about the life or temperament of each one of them. Then in her eagerness to have me get acquainted with my town she would go on to tell me life histories of various other Castine characters who came into her mind because of their queerness or their tragedy or their comicalness. Then after that, as our absorbing conversations progressed day after day that first autumn, she went on to tell me about her own family, about her three brothers and her one sister and their lives. I loved to listen to her. Sometimes when she talked about people there was a suppressed intensity of feeling in her voice. Often she couldn't seem to keep pity out of it or indignation. Most of all she couldn't suppress something that seemed to trouble her continually, and that was the question of why such terrible things had to happen to people's lives.

The thing that struck me as I listened to her was the loneliness of her mind. Nobody else around her thought about things the way she did, with deep passionate concern. And the curious tremor in her rich, strong voice when she talked intimately to me made me suspect that this was the first time she had ever spoken her thoughts aloud to anyone. When it was my turn I told her about my own family and friends and their lives. My effort to describe them to her made them all come vividly and dramatically into my mind, set off against the background of the little kitchen, and I grew very elated when I saw them all in my mind's eye, arriving there the following summer in a grand bustle of eagerness to see and admire my house, and to enter with me the great new era in our lives which I believed was to be started there. I could see them walking on the brick path, or sitting on the terrace around a tea table, and glancing up, saying, "Is that Mount Desert that we see over there? And where is Ile au Haut from here?" They all looked so delightful and so interesting to me in my mind's eye that I longed to show them to Lorna and to have her know them. I tried to describe them in such a way that they would look as interesting to her as they did to me. I told her about my artistic and literary friends, and in describing to her their characters and experiences and wanderings I felt as if I were describing something as brilliant and romantic and mad as the court life in some exotic foreign country. This was partly because she was such a wonderful listener, for she put as much intentness and ardor into hearing my stories as she did into telling me her own.

When I told her how eager I was to have her know my friends and my family and to have them know her I could not help showing a little of my private opinion as to the impression she would make on them. It gave me pleasure to anticipate what I thought would be a novel and exciting experience for her, that of being recognized and appreciated for the person she really was, a person of unusual qualities and beauty. I knew that friends

108

of mine like Catharine Huntington and Eleanor Clement would meet her without that barrier which she was accustomed to feel between herself and people from the city. But when I tried to say anything to her about how much my friends would admire her and like to know her she recoiled as if I had said something grotesque.

"What would they want to know a thing like me for?" she would say. "No! I'll come and see you when you're alone, but not when there's company. Why, I wouldn't know what to say to people like that. What could I say that they'd want to hear? Just a plain humdrum thing like me—I haven't got an idea in my head."

"But just be natural," I would plead, "the way you are with me. That is what they like best and they're always hunting for it. They will think you are beautiful, too, the same as I do . . . because you are, really."

"Oh, my goodness me! Me beautiful—!"

Her laughter would peal forth again. Her laughter startled me because it suddenly made me realize how rarely I had ever heard boisterous laughter that made a beautiful sound. Hers was like a handful of bells, shaken vigorously, once, twice, three times or more, making a delicious hypnotizing cascade of sound. There was nothing to do for a minute but listen and delight in it. There was no use to argue.

She was always stubbornly humorous whenever I tried to make her understand how rare she was. She refused to be impressed by anything I said about her. She would not budge one inch from her idea of the kind of person she was and what she was good for. I had to yield to her baffling laughter and try not to bother any more about what she might be missing and what all the others were missing who didn't know her and never would, with her consent.

At noon and at suppertime her husband came home. His name was Alvah. He was an unreflective, boyish person, a tall, big, blue-eyed young carpenter in blue overalls. As soon as he came home he would lean over the washbasin in the kitchen washing his hands and face. Sometimes he would turn his head away from the mirror where he was combing his hair to tell us something funny he had heard, with a whimsical little boy's smile, or to laugh at one of our stories.

They had never had a boarder before, and I was afraid at first that Alvah, although he had consented to doing it, might not enjoy having their privacy invaded. In spite of his boyishness and amiability, a certain dignity and aloofness came over him at times which frightened me. Sometimes I caught a look of rather cold shrewdness in his blue eyes as if he were sizing me up. So I found myself trying humbly to make him like me by being the little clown. I discovered it pleased him to hear ridiculous things about the summer people. I could always make him laugh by telling about Mary, and quoting her and describing some of the absurd, childish, rebellious jokes she had played on people. In the beginning it seemed to me that Alvah laughed immoderately at these stories as if he saw more in them than I did, and I felt a horrified suspicion that I was paying my way by making other people and perhaps Mary ridiculous in a way I had not intended. I suddenly thought I could hear my private little stories being passed around with loud guffaws among

Alvah and his cronies. But I decided that this, if true, was only fair. None of the innocent absurdities concerning the summer people which I could hand over to the townspeople to enjoy could ever equal the number of funny stories about the townspeople, already collected and treasured and passed around by the bright, literary summer people who had been slyly at it for years.

This unexpected rapport provided our mealtimes with really great hilarity and gave us a feeling of warm joyous sympathy toward each other. I would tell some idiotic little story about a summer person, and in return they would tell me a story making one of the village people ridiculous, which had for me the same extra content of absurdity that mine had for them. The fact that we were all so generously exchanging and betraying our friends right and left made us all three laugh until we cried. Alvah must have been six feet tall, or more, and his laughter was in proportion to his size. The first terrific explosions seemed as if they would split the woodwork and break the walls; then as he gasped and groaned I used to be almost afraid to look at him. Lorna's blackbirdlike throat poured out a laughing aria, and as for me the tears streamed down and I ached and was frightened.

When Alvah with a final sigh of exhaustion said good-by to us after dinner and went back to work, or in the evening to his Lodge meetings, Lorna and I would turn again to our old wives' tales. Neither of us ever grew tired or indifferent to anything the other had to say, whether it was funny or contemplative. When we were alone we usually fell instinctively into the sober, wondering mood which

111

seemed to be the natural climate of us both. When people share that particular attitude they never tire of each other. And as this attitude is one which is usually hidden, locked up inside year upon end for lack of anyone who shares it, such people are usually lonely people who never get over the miracle of having found somebody, if they ever do, who shares it.

But sooner or later in the midst of our conversations, if it were still daylight, I would feel an overwhelming desire to go to my house. Lorna always watched me go with ardent sympathy. She liked the way I felt about my house, and she never minded having our conversations interrupted for its sake. I was like a person who is in love, and Lorna understood and let me go my way, as a good friend always will. A sudden feeling would come over me and I just had to go. My eagerness to know my house was even greater than my eagerness to know my neighbors. After all, that was why I was there.

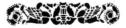

18.

AS soon as I set foot on my land I would stand still and look all around. I would drift a little way and then go motionless as a rock, staring like an idiot. And I would like to tell about some of the things that impressed me first. One of my new treasures which attracted my attention in the beginning was the brick path along the front of the house. It was an old brick path laid in the grass leading in from the road to my front door—a door which had a fanlight above it in whose thin old glass the light of the sea was reflected. I had been brought up in a city famous for its Georgian architecture, where fanlights and brick garden paths are found even in the slums. I had been brought up never to pass any beautiful specimen of our architecture without noticing it and admiring it. And yet our family happened never to have owned or lived in one of those Georgian houses. I could not believe at first that I myself now possessed a fanlight and a brick path, and not even in the slums or the too familiar and respectable streets of Salem, but surrounded by the enhancing light and air of a town where I was alone and free.

My predecessor had evidently not valued his brick path and he had ignored it for so long that the grass had reached over it from both sides until only the middle bricks were visible. I got Mr. Austen Bowden, the gardener, to come and cut the turf away and uncover all the bricks again. They were pink and purple and blue, and in my opinion they were extremely beautiful. Mr. Bowden found and uncovered also another branch of the path which went beyond the front door to the far corner of the dooryard. This branch had been buried not only under the grass but under the rugosa rose bushes that spread over it from the bed in front of the south sitting-room windows. After the whole path had been uncovered and restored I used to walk to the far end of it and I felt as if I were walking on a captain's walk, because at the far end the land dropped away and the path seemed to jut out high above the harbor.

I used to stand there feeling like a proud captain high on my brick path and stare humbly at the wonderful things in front of me, at the great fortune that had come to me, the dark islands and the turquoise water and the lilting motion of the Brooksville hills.

Those things were all strange and new to me that first autumn, so that I did not see them as a whole but separately. I could not see them with the same eyes as I did afterward when I had looked at them so many times that at last they became fused in an inevitable whole. The curious magic of repetition molded them together at last until they made something complete in itself, like a phrase of music, in which not a note could have been changed without destroying its meaning and its power over me.

After I had stared my fill from the path I would walk around onto the terrace behind the house. There I found another lovely door and a smooth granite doorstep to admire and to sit on. I would twist around to look up at the door while I sat on the stone. It was an old heavy one—its panels made a beautifully proportioned cross. There were fluted pilasters on each side and across the top four bubbly panes of glass. It opened out of a little square entry between the kitchen and the south sitting room.

Sitting on the comfortable warm stone I looked down across my field. Along the southern boundary a row of balm of Gilead trees made a thin screen through which I could see the roofs and chimneys of the houses down on Water Street, against the blue river. At the eastern end of the screen my land turned a corner and went in a long strip down to the water front where it ended on the beach among the fishermen's shacks. Even out in the water I owned property. My wreck was out there. If you rowed out at low tide you could look down through the water and see it, I was told. It was a historical wreck, the British transport *St. Helena* which had been sunk in 1778 by American guns firing on her from Nautilus Island opposite. I was told about it first by a man named Frank Grindle whom I had hired to paint the outside of the house. Mr. Douglas told me he was very quick and wouldn't charge as much as some of the other painters. He had an eager, nervous face, and he was a great talker. When he came down off his ladder he used to stop and talk with me, and one day he told me I owned a wreck. He said he'd often been out in his dory and reached down and got pieces of wood off her, old oak that had been so long in the water that it was as hard as a rock and black as ebony after it was carved into something and oiled and polished. Several people owned carved chairs and other things that had been made out of it. One day when he came to work he brought me one of his pieces of my wreck. He promised he would take me out in his dory at what he called the next low dreen of tide so that I might look down and see the half-buried vessel for myself.

I liked Frank Grindle because when he first began to talk to me his eyes shone with witty amusement at the idea of my being the proprietor of the *St. Helena*, and because he seemed to know it would amuse me too. He used to talk very fast and eagerly about other things besides—all kinds of things—and while he was talking his eyes would dwell on me with an attentive, indulgent, smiling look, somewhat as if I were a child. He told me things about himself.

He told me he had been around the world, working on what he always called palace yachts, one time with a Vanderbilt and again with an Astor. That was where he learned manners, he said, and he spoke disparagingly of the bad manners he thought I would probably notice in most of the other men in town who had never been out in the world and had never learned, he said, the proper way to address a lady. He told me that after he came home from sea he got to drinking so he was drunk and a disgrace all the time, and how he had cured himself by going into the Maine woods as a lumberman and how he had hurt his thumb in the woods and amputated it himself because there was no doctor there. Very proudly he made me look at the stump so I could see what a neat job he had done. With a grin he even told me male things which would ordinarily have made me feel very shy and embarrassed. But he had a different attitude toward me from any man I had known before. There was something essentially courteous about him which I do not think he had had to learn from the Vanderbilts or the Astors, something which made everything he said or did seem natural and good. I had not yet learned that everybody in that amazing, liberated town took it for granted that every adult, married or not, was a fully experienced human being in love, even if they were not so experienced in education or manners, which require special advantages.

I asked Lorna if Frank Grindle's stories were true. For in spite of his candor there was something extravagant and unbelievable about him. She declared that strange as they did sound they were true. He had been a terrible drunkard and since he cured himself he had never drunk again. He was a great reader as well as a talker, she said. He took four or five books a week out of the library. He liked books about science. Everybody in town believed that if he had had an education he would have been somebody. I could believe that too. There was something magnetic in his eagerness. With education he might have had a very different kind of life. I felt guilty toward him because of my own advantages, and because he was a gifted man who lacked advantages and was scarcely conscious of it, content to live out his life with his gifts undeveloped in a kind of childish obscurity.

Frank Grindle played a part in the beginning of my life there, and he played a part very near the end. After I had lived in my house several summers he told me one day how glad he always was to see the lights in my windows the first night I came back in the spring. He liked a pink lamp shade which he could see from his house at the bottom of the field. It made a rosy light, he said, and it was nice to see it after the house had stood up there dark and empty all winter. One spring morning, the next to the last year that I came back there, as I was driving along the road from Bucksport toward Castine, I was anticipating my arrival and, among all the other familiar things deliciously reawakening in my mind as I came nearer and nearer, I was thinking of how Frank Grindle would probably be pleased to see the rosy lamp that night. The first piece of news I heard as I stepped out of my car was that he had been killed an hour before. He had always been too impatient, too quick, people said, and didn't take time enough to make his staging solid, and that morning

117

he had just gone up on it to paint the eaves of the Castine Inn when the staging gave way and he was killed the instant he struck the ground.

The thought of him has interrupted my attempt to describe my house and land. For when I think of the first autumn, and remember myself sitting on the terrace doorstep meditating about the *St. Helena,* I cannot help remembering Frank Grindle too, and how he spoke and smiled. He was so alive that he is even now more vivid to me than any of the other men who worked for me at the same time—men who are still living and whom I see occasionally, still going about their business, getting a little oldish, a little grayish, and putting on spectacles when they work. That first autumn his ladder was always somewhere up against the house and he was slapping thick, white paint onto the clapboards, while I sat at a lower altitude on the terrace doorstep, enjoying the warm sense of unspoken friendship and protection surrounding me.

From the terrace my exploring gaze as it traveled slowly round my boundaries moved eastward from the strip of beach, which was scarcely visible through the balm of Gileads and the little houses between, among them Frank Grindle's, and then came slowly up the eastern slope where I saw filling the whole horizon on my left the old leaning willows that marked the northeastern boundary.

I have always loved willows, because they are the only trees who have wantonly escaped from the classic idea of a tree; because instead of growing straight up into the air they lean sideways at all sorts of sad and desperate angles, their branches jutting out of them anywhere, like soft green spray, instead of being placed symmetrically on each side of the trunk, and because sometimes even four or five trunks grow fanwise out of one root. This waywardness in their structure gives willows a look of wild romantic abandon, as though they were changelings and held the spirits of people who have been crossed in love. I like them, too, because they can be so old, all tumble-down and rotten and apparently dead, and yet when April comes there will rise out of those black, crumbling ruins the most tender and youthful green wands, holding new leaves high in the air in great, round, soft, billowy bouquets, more expressive of spring than any other tree. Because of this wonderful mingling of agedness and tender youth willows seem to belong to a race of trees apart, one that is ancient and magic and lorn. I felt very rich and lucky indeed as I stared at my own row of willows arching down the slope. Their shapes made a wonderful decorated border against the eastern sky, of whirls and scallops and festoons, which my eyes were never to grow tired of tracing.

Just in front of the willows stood a little weather-beaten building, which I always made sure to include in each of my roaming, exploring, appreciative glances round my place. My glance not only included it without fail but always stopped for a moment or longer to give a special secret caressing thought to it, and a promise for the future. I had not forgotten that when the idea of buying a house first struck me I had believed that I wanted to buy a thimble, and nothing but a thimble—that is, a small weather-beaten outbuilding or cluster of outbuildings which I would transform into something fas-

cinating on a doll-size scale. Afterward, when to my
surprise I had bought a large and very real house
on a grand scale, again to my surprise I discovered
that I had also bought a thimble, without even knowing it. For, along with my house, land, brick path,
fanlight, willows, and historical wreck—along with
all these magnificent, incredible treasures—a thimble
had been thrown in free. And a perfect thimble.

It was no mere ramshackle old shed, but a solid
well-proportioned little building, containing one
room with six windows and two doors, and a loft
above the room. I was told by my neighbors that it
had originally been a creamhouse. Later it had been
used as a henhouse, but for a long time it had not
been used at all. Inside, when I first looked in, was
as uninviting as an ex-henhouse is likely to be. The
half-open loft appeared to be stuffed with old boards
and dust and cobwebs, but the dark beams were
sound and the lower floor was firm and strong. After
it had been thoroughly washed and scrubbed a good
many times I discovered that the floor of the thimble
was particularly beautiful, made as it was of very
wide, old boards, curiously rich in color, mottled
and stained from use and age until they had become a deep purplish brown, blending into purplish
gray and dark brown.

After I had the rickety loft torn down and cleared
away, the room was almost square and open to the
peaked roof. I had the walls whitewashed and put
in a Franklin stove, a low bench, a wicker settee,
and an old stand-up desk painted blue which I
found on the premises. After the loft was gone the
light which came in from a square window in the
western gable of the loft and the light from the four

other windows made the old creamhouse all I could possibly have dreamed of in a thimble.

It is the beautiful purplish boards in the floors which I remember now with a peculiar vividness and intimacy of feeling, because I used so often later on to stare at and admire them in vacant spellbound pauses while I was writing in the thimble, lying on a low wicker settee only a few inches higher than the floor. For during the summers of my life there I became the inhabitant of the thimble for several hours each day. It was my close-fitting, protecting shell which held only me alone; I was the little, soft, amorphous, silent one who lived inside it, like a snail, and almost grew to be a part of it during those hours. When I was writing I tended to become my original shell-less, impressionable, unguarded self, the unworldly child of God who exists inside of every person, more or less imprisoned; and it was therefore necessary to acquire a shell such as my thimble for protection during those hours when one took off the protection of the outer self. Toward a sanctuary of this kind, or I suppose toward any sanctuary which shelters the spirit and allows it to be free, a love develops which has a quality of deep and intimate gratitude. This grateful love can only be felt toward a room or a house in which one spends many hours alone, for just as soon as a dwelling is shared by two or more people that intimacy is impaired. Even the best and closest human relationship will at times drive the spirit into a corner where it sits, a bewildered and forlorn captive.

When I was in my thimble, and in this impressionable state, I used to be aware of other living but nonhuman inhabitants who shared my shell with me.

121

They were silent as I was, or their voices were too small to hear. Against those deep-purplish boards one morning I watched in shocked horror the convulsions of a chalk-white butterfly being carefully strangled by a spider, after it had flown into the web and caught its wings. I watched the spider clasp the butterfly until it shook in the orgasm of death, and its wings drooped and did not move again. The spider kept on handling it, turning it over and over on his thread until it had ceased to have any resemblance to a butterfly and was only a narrow little bundle left hanging in the web; and then the spider skated off passing by on his way another little dried package, the corpse of an earlier victim, and then disappeared under a columbine leaf outside the open door.

Almost every morning in summer when I opened the thimble door I heard a buzzing sound and found bees inside the yellow tin lantern which hung from the ceiling, and I had to struggle with them to show them the way out to freedom. The lantern was a present from my cousins, the Robsons; and when Henry Beston came on a visit at my house the first summer he made a great ceremonial business of hanging it up for me in my thimble. He went to the Dennett Brothers' ship chandlery on Dennett's wharf and bought some rope and a brass cleat and a pulley, and he rigged the lantern up in a highly nautical style, so that it would hang from the beam in the middle of the room and I could raise or lower it by the rope attached to the pulley. It happened that the top of the lantern had a fluted edge which made several small entrances into its interior that nobody would ever have noticed except the amorous bees who evidently notice all such entrances. For all the bees who came near the thimble on summer days mistook the lantern for a flower and they crawled through the attractive little openings and then could not find their way out again. Almost every morning when I arrived I heard their angry, impatient rumbling and I quickly lowered the lantern and opened its hinged door and urged them to realize quickly that they were free. Sometimes even on sharp fall mornings, when I came and had to build a fire in the stove before I could begin to work, there were bees in the lantern and they were cold, lying still in the bottom around the candle socket as if they were dead. As the room warmed up from the fire inside and the sun on the roof they would begin to waken, and after they had got their bearings they would sail out into the mellowing autumn day.

There was one more of these nonhuman persons who came into my thimble. A hummingbird darted in one day and flew up into the peaked roof, high above the windows and the open door by which he had come in. He flew back and forth, and back and forth, in what appeared to be a kind of frenzy of terror. I opened every window and both doors, hoping to show him that he too was free to go. He was flying high above my reach and I watched helplessly. It seemed a pity that he couldn't see what was so simple. Finally I left him, thinking that he might do better if he were alone. When I came back several hours later he was gone. At last he had made the great discovery that what he had imagined was a prison was really open wide.

My thimble, I adored it! I planted morning-glory vines that grew up on strings over the outside. I used to look up from my work and see blue or purple silk morning-glories trembling against the edge of a window in the sun. Sometimes I used to feel and hear a brisk little wind suddenly seize the thimble in its clutch, and knock the vines against the outside walls; then the capricious little Castine wind would go away as suddenly as it had come and leave the thimble and its inhabitants in our usual stillness.

From my terrace doorstep, like the three sections of a Japanese screen, I saw on my left the willows and the thimble, in the middle the balm of Gileads and the fishermen's houses and the Bay and the islands, and over on my right I saw my neighbors' place, the Douglas house and barn and orchard and henhouse and manure heap. It was not a picturesque group of farm buildings. They were not old enough. The long clapboarded blank wall of the barn was a depressing object and it blocked out a large piece of the southwest horizon. But I liked it. I didn't want to insist that everything in sight should be beautiful. I liked my neighbors' place. The sun poured down all day long on this southern slope of ours, and I was glad that at least one of us worked on it and made it fruitful. I liked the sounds that came from the Douglas place, the sunny cry of a rooster in the morning and the hens clucking and the rattle of the milk cans. I liked the moment in the late afternoon when Mr. Douglas brought his cows home from pasture. His three Jersey cows wore sweet-sounding bells each of a different note, and as they came along the road toward the house at four o'clock every afternoon their bells would suddenly come within earshot. As the three cows came nearer, swinging slowly along from side to side, the three bells grew louder and mingled unevenly in a kind of haphazard melody that was rich and sweet in the stillness. It reached its sudden crescendo when they came into sight and crossed the road, and then as quickly it was extinguished as one by one they disappeared into the barn. It would have been beautiful to hear their bells at daybreak when they went out and away up the road, but I never heard them then because I was always deep asleep at that hour.

Because my neighbors' day began and ended so much earlier than mine our two cycles of consciousness did not coincide at many points. And they were too busy to pay any attention to me. I got a nod and an affectionate smile from Mrs. Douglas and a cheerful shout from him and a friendly wave of the hand, if his hands were not too full, whenever we happened to see each other from our respective domains. They were perpetually busy. I would see her stepping with her quick little footsteps in and out of her henyard, and I would see him swinging a pitchfork or carrying squashes in from the autumn garden or bringing in his full milk pails at night. I knew I did not need to fear that I would ever be intruded upon or disturbed by neighbors whose life consisted of such an endless round of work as theirs.

I felt proud of my neighbors because of the way their life contrasted with the life of the summer people. They had useful feet and legs that carried them around all day, their hands knew how to deal with fundamental things, with the ground and seeds and tools and animals. I knew that if I had had summer cottagers next door our overstimulated brains and our useless hands and feet would have contrived to build up between us an elaborate awareness of each other from which there would be no rest. When I saw the Douglases going about their business, looking so refreshingly unaware of themselves and of me, I knew that I could go about my business with the same freedom as they did for all they would ever notice or care. With them for neighbors I had hit upon a combination which to me has always seemed too good to be true, the combination of personal freedom and physical coziness. For while I rejoiced in feeling so wonderfully free and unnoticed on my doorstep I also felt relaxed and comfortable because if I wanted them they were near, so competent and friendly. There can even be something wonderful in the smell of a manure pile when it is carried on the crystal air of the North Atlantic seacoast. When the wind brought a whiff of that rich country smell to me from the Douglas barnyard on those autumn days it gave me a feeling of utter satisfaction concerning my neighbors.

Our joint solitude, the Douglases' and mine, was interrupted now and then throughout the day by the moving profile of someone going up or down the right of way. Before I signed the deed Judge Patterson had told me about this footpath along the edge of my land. It was mentioned in the deed and he wanted to be sure that I understood that people using it were not trespassing but going where they had a right to go. Sometimes I would see an anxious-looking little girl slipping hurriedly along the path, leading a smaller child by the hand; or a boy alone wearing a hunting cap and carrying a gun. Sometimes a man with a massive chest and shoulders, who, they told me, was Ed Brigham, went swinging down the path at noon on his way home to dinner.

I enjoyed seeing those quiet passers-by. They almost never looked around, but kept their eyes down on the path or straight ahead. When they appeared usually one at a time, and curved along the little arc of the hillside and then disappeared again, they seemed like symbolical figures, each representing a certain human quality, one the unconscious pathos of a motherly little girl and another a boy's secret lusty adventurousness. They all used their legal right to pass across my land with such diffidence and modesty that their intent profiles seemed only to give accent to the solitude that lay around me.

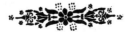

19

THERE were two other things I noticed and marveled at in my new world. One of these was the sun and the other was the air. I had never seen a world so gilded and so richly bathed and blessed by such a benign sun as that world was by that sun. The sun seemed to pour down a lavish, golden, invulnerable contentment on everything, on people, houses, animals, fields—and a sweetness like the sweetness of passion. The sun had so much room to shine in there. It had the whole sky to shine in, and it had miles and miles of hills and woods, it had islands and rocks and boats to glisten on and soak into like oil. And it was thanks to the matchless air of that peninsula that such a flood of sunshine never became a burden. It always seemed exactly right, golden and voluptuous yet without weight. It was as if the air there were so buoyant that it always lifted up part of the weight of the sun's heat and kept it from ever falling too heavily on our shoulders. It was indescribable air. It made every day seem like a gala day. We never woke up to an ordinary humdrum morning.

I noticed these two things, the air and the sun, at my own house more than I had ever noticed them at the other end of the town. I imagined that the reason for this was that my house responded to sun and air more than most houses do. Sometimes it felt like a boat at anchor. There is that curious quality about all the little noises on a boat which makes them sound unmistakably boaty. The tapping of a rope against canvas, the squeak of a pulley, a voice or a footstep heard on a boat are different from the same sounds heard on land. They are magnified and yet softened by the sea air. All such little noises around my house struck me as having that same soft boaty sound. A clothespin dropped on the doorstep had it, and the rustle of a curtain in an open window sounded like a sail fluttering. When the window sill burned my fingers on a hot morning it was just as if I had touched the gunwale of a dory that had been lying in the sun for hours.

They were so compelling, the divine air and the brilliant sun on my doorstep and all around me as far as I could see, that I stopped thinking. They made thinking seem ridiculous. The thing that would have been the most natural thing to do was to change into a plant or a fruit tree, and I almost felt myself changing. There was no other way to express my thanks for all this, except to burst into leaves and flowers.

The Little Locksmith

Until I might be able to achieve such expression the fullness of my joy was sometimes too painful to bear, simply because it was too big to be contained inside my chest. Then in order to dissipate it I would get up and move around. I would go inside the house and watch Mr. Gardner and his helper building the new fireplace in the southwest sitting room where my predecessor had torn it out, because he was not a fireplace man. It would have relieved me a little if I could have seen something that disappointed me; but even when I discovered, too late to change it, that one side of the new fireplace was not quite straight I couldn't really mind. Imperfection and perfection were both included in the universe and I had good reason to make friends with imperfection. Besides it was impossible for me to be displeased with Mr. Gardner. He was such a gentle soft-spoken man and he was proud of his trade of masonry. His wife's sister was a nursemaid in my brother's family in Salem. Jonny and Harriet had spent a summer with their nurse at Mr. Gardner's house and had concocted, at the ages of three and four, a large boat in his back yard. He used to act protectively toward me too, like Frank Grindle.

After I had stood and watched him I would cross the wide hall and admire the graceful staircase, and from there I would go into the west sitting room and through the passage into the big country dining room whose woodwork and cupboard and mantelpiece were painted a countrified mustard yellow that I liked very much. I would roam through the huge kitchen and the pantries and then up the back stairs, with many long pauses and imaginings in the large square bedrooms, and I would gloat over the interesting queer long narrow bathroom whose window looked down over the harbor. After that I would climb up into the attic where there were four more bedrooms and a wide hall with one dormer window from which I could see farther down the bay than from any other place in the house. From the windows of the east rooms in the attic on clear days I would stare at the pale-blue bubble that they had told me was Mount Desert, and at the azure cone for which the town of Blue Hill is named. Since there was not a chair and not even a box to sit down on in any room of the house I would presently roam down the attic stairs again and open the paneled door that led from the shadowy back hall to the lightness and gaiety and elegance of the front hall, the fanlight, and the wide, graceful, easy stairs. Feeling assuaged and calmed from my little exercise, I would go down the lovely shallow stairs and out onto the front doorstep to sit again until my satisfaction had accumulated once more to an uncomfortable size.

On the front doorstep I used to quiet my soaring spirits by leaning over to watch the crickets walking on the bricks. I found there was another right of way not mentioned in the deed. The largest, handsomest, glossiest crickets I had ever seen were traveling up and down on the newly uncovered pink and purple bricks. It was the season and the weather that crickets love. I knew that they were one of the best possible signs of good luck to a house, and when one of them walked in over the doorsill and through the front door to utter a loud resounding chirp in the hall I knew that all would be well. In appreciation of this omen I decided, as though I were a royal personage, that I would have a cricket embroidered on all the linen that was to be used in the house.

I began to have all kinds of flowery ideas. As I bent over and watched the crickets I felt a kind of medieval delight toward them, like the delight which must have been felt by the makers of tapestries and moved them to weave into the corners of their great scenes the smallest insects and birds, field flowers and trees in bud, and graceful little animals. The treasure that had come into my hands waked in me a new warmth of perception and love toward everything I saw. It stirred the need to give adornment and value to every detail of the life to be lived there. As in a medieval embroidery I wanted everything to be included, I wanted the humorous and the romantic, the marvelous and the quaint, the grand and the humble, the wild and the gentle, all to be brought together there in a hymn of praise. I and my estate were in microcosm like people and their country just arrived at a rich, leisured period in their history when the people began to express their happiness by adorning their daily lives in a thousand ways, bringing forth a period in their history during which the decorative arts flourish. In every country there seems to be at least one such period of worship and thanks, a time so happy that everything the hands of its people touch becomes a work of art.

In humility and elation I felt that I had arrived at such a period, and that I was an instrument being used to bring such a period into the history of my family. For I hoped that this house might be a magnet that would attract them all and especially the six children who represented in our family then the new generation. I wanted my house to be used as a cradle for such great magnetic things as art and writing and science—indeed, for the shelter and nourishment of the human spirit in any of those many different yet interchangeable forms in which it delights to manifest itself. I wanted my house filled to overflowing with all the necessary materials to awaken and sustain the rich life of the imagination and the intellect; I wanted it filled with paints and pencils and drawing paper, canvas and crayons, heaps of beautiful books piled up everywhere, reproductions of drawings, art magazines and literary reviews, maps, musical instruments and books of music, a microscope, a compass, and a great globe of the world, a telescope, and books about astronomy, about geology, about shells, insects, and birds, and I wanted all kinds of games, packs of cards, a checker board, chessmen, dice and dominoes.

And I wanted to think of a name for my house, to be embroidered underneath the cricket. I hoped I could think of a name which would attach itself to the house by a natural affinity and would be forever connected with it in everybody's mind. Whatever the name might turn out to be I thought of its acquiring such associations through summer after summer that it would become a unique, beloved name in our family, just as the name Stowe had been loved and adored by us in our childhood. I found the letter about crickets in White's *Natural History of Selborne*, and I was enchanted with their Latin name, Grylla. Grylla Farm, I thought, tentatively—Grylla House; Grylla was rather a funny-sounding word, but it might become a nice one, I thought, if it were used and made familiar. But I needed to try it for a little while to find out if it was right, and in the meantime because in all the long exuberant letters that I wrote on my knee from the doorstep to my family and friends I burst into ecstasies so many times about the crickets and the brick path, they were amused at me and one of them made up the pseudo-Welsh name Cricket-y-brick, which they adopted and always used because they thought it was cute and sounded like me.

But I didn't want a cute name for my sober, grand, romantic house, the house which I thought of as an expression of my rebellion against cuteness. I wanted room here to be something else than the cunning little De La Mare character, room to find out what I really was, and room to be whatever I really was. I had boldly seized a piece of the earth to grow on, and had instantly taken root. Everything I looked at fed my will to do now the things I had always quietly believed in but had never done. In this divine situation I could begin at last. I could begin to live.

And so a kind of mystic marriage, an impregnation, took place between me and that piece of land and the buildings that stood on it. And it was a happy marriage. From the moment when I first stepped onto those premises until the last moment when I left them I felt a presence there, a strong, loving spirit that was always brooding over me, welcoming me and encouraging me. I knew from the feeling of it that that place had been at some time or other blessed in some mysterious way, and was particularly cherished and guarded by the gods. I felt an influence on me there that was beyond explanation, as if the rays of all my good stars had met above the roof, thanks to some almost unheard-of mathematical harmony; and that they made an invisible graph, or diagram, a kind of cat's cradle or snow-crystal design of good fortune, and were being held there, caught in perpetual balance. Certain places are fond of certain people, and I am sure that place was fond of me. But I wasn't the only person who felt its benign influence. Nearly everybody who came there felt it too. There was something about my place, a kind of unusual glow and a warmth over it, which seemed at moments to give us the feeling of an almost immortal happiness. I have never had that feeling in any other place.

I didn't realize all that at first. I knew from the beginning that the house was my friend and my ally, and after I had sat on the doorstep during those first long Indian summer days I began to know that it was going to be my Magna Carta. And I began to make bold plans, in obedience to the mysterious will which had brought me there. Having obeyed it once, I now felt the desire for action really waking and moving about in me.

And since the story I have to tell is the story of the working out of those bold plans I will have to pause now long enough to tell what the plans were, and why they expressed things which had waited and been shut up in me so long. There was a certain naïveté about my plans, and therefore they did not work out as I expected, which is all the more reason for telling what they were in the beginning, because in their working out they became almost unrecognizable.

134

20

I BELIEVED passionately that every human being could be happy. I believed that everybody should pursue his own kind of happiness boldly and positively. Because I happened to have been deprived of what is generally considered necessary for a happy life, I had used all my wits to circumvent my fate, to make something out of nothing. I believed I had discovered in this process a few valuable tricks to outwit fate with, tricks by which I myself had got hold of a most extraordinary joy. My particular kind of joy happened to come through the medium of writing. Because in the midst of the bewilderments of my youth it was that particular door in my mind which I had stumbled upon and escaped through into bliss, it was the writer's medium which I had learned to know. There were certain conditions necessary to the full experience of that kind of happiness and these I believed I understood and was qualified to establish and to offer in my house. There were also two other kinds of happiness which I believed I understood. I wanted to use my house to provide these three kinds of opportunity for fulfillment, not only for myself, but for any others who wanted them.

My first discovery of the bliss I could experience in writing had happened long before. And when I first discovered that door in my mind I found also that I could not always open it when I wanted to, especially if I wanted to very badly indeed. But after a period of struggle and despair I hit upon an abracadabra which almost never failed to open the door for me. Once safe inside, I worked like a spider, secretly and alone. The only tools I required were a pencil and a block of paper and solitude. Also, for its safety, this joy required a certain kind of understanding and protection on the part of others. This I had never really got, and I wanted a chance to demonstrate it and to give it myself to people like me who needed it.

For although the happiness came out of me like the thread out of a spider, its continued existence was dependent on protection from outside things. It was always in danger of being injured or altogether thwarted, because daily human life is not designed to recognize and guard this curious happiness. Cloisters and monasteries were invented in order to protect the life of the spirit from the life of the world, and any young person who in modern times tries to live the life of the spirit without protection is almost sure to come to grief. When in my case the life of the spirit was injured or thwarted or even threatened I suffered, it seemed, out of all reason. I felt as if a storm or an earthquake had struck my psyche. All of a sudden I felt destroyed, horribly defeated. All life seemed torn to pieces.

Usually this panic of frustration came from a temporary interruption of my working hours caused by personal demands on me which I could not refuse without betraying my own loving and responsible instincts as a human being. Perhaps the reason why my family's encroachments tortured me so much was because they were all so fond and loving, and yet they seemed to emphasize the absence in my life of the one personal demand canceling all others which is the cry of youth. I was trying to kill my sense of loss in that direction by giving myself with equal passion to the life of the spirit. But I lived in the midst of an affectionate charming family, and I am sure that there is no greater obstacle to a person who is just beginning to be a writer.

I had never heard any discussion of the eternal irreconcilability between the dedicated life and the personal life. But underneath the surface of the small encroachments of my secret life by the people I loved and who loved me I could intuitively feel the existence of a fundamental conflict; and it terrified me because I knew that if I should ever have to face that conflict and if I should fail to defend successfully my right to pursue this life of dedication I should perish. My self, the vital part of me, the precious joy I had discovered, would cease to exist. Although every serious person is expected to feel a responsibility toward his work as well as toward the people he loves, there is a point beyond which his devotion to his work cannot go without arousing the antagonism and jealousy of the people who love him and whom he loves. And as everyone knows, Art is jealous too. This conflict can be as tragic as a civil war, because it is a war of the heart, between people who love each other.

I think perhaps it is a religious war. I am sure that my solitary brooding and writing were a form of worship. I believed that romantic love, if I could have experienced it, would have been a form of worship. Since I was denied that form I had found this lonelier way of expressing my feeling of passionate adoration toward the mystery of life. And just as a young person preparing himself for a religious life must train himself rigorously before he is able to pursue his meditations at regular hours and for any length of time without fatigue or inattention, I had to train myself in my chosen form of devotion before I was capable of giving myself up to it every day for longer and longer periods. Sometimes when I went into my room in the morning I went toward my table with loathing. I hated the little heap of pages, the pencils, the block of paper. They seemed like horrid medicine that was being forced on me. I was very young when I began and my youth rebelled against the unnatural solitude and inactivity and discipline of such a life. But I knew that for me there was no other way. It was only by that particular discipline that I could ever find any path for the mysterious feelings of rebellion and desire that tortured me so. I felt as if half of me was an eager, high-spirited army on prancing horses, all on fire to explore and conquer a rich and unknown land, but held in check on the border because there was no road by which it could enter. And half of me was a division of humble slaves put at work to build the road over which the army could ride. The pain and patience and slow precision needed to build the road were evenly balanced by the fiery impatience of the restive army.

I would sit down at my table with this conflict raging in me. I could use my will to get myself to the table and to keep myself sitting there, but I soon learned that I could not use my will to get myself any farther along. The next thing I learned was that I must lay aside my will. I must depend on the patient humble slaves. I taught myself to sit perfectly still, in passive acquiescent obedience, waiting for whatever was to come. I began to realize at last the important truth, that I, or any other writer or artist, must always remain a humble servant and never assume the part of arrogant master. The prancing army was not me. I was only the one who patiently built the road over which it might ride. As soon as I grasped this my turbulence and my egotistical despair and my will subsided. I learned to be inexhaustibly patient, utterly submissive. At last, after I was able to arrive at this state almost every day, making my mind empty and receptive, my reward would be granted to me. Beginning gradually and imperceptibly the way sleep comes, something would begin to happen on the paper in front of me. The people in my story would begin to move. The place they were in, the rooms, the house, would come alive before me, opening like a flower, mysterious, ravishing. I listened and watched with swiftly mounting excitement and fascination until suddenly it was no longer possible for me to restrain my hand from seizing the pencil.

Until I had striven for humility I could do nothing at all. Therefore it hurt me bitterly to find that in order to make a barricade around the necessary time and solitude within which to serve my religion I had to make myself seem to be anything but humble. I had to let myself be thought conceited and self-centered and ruthless, thus hurting and bewildering not only the people who loved me, but hurting and bewildering my own social and human self as well. I knew that I was not conceited and ruthless. It was only an accident that made me need to appear so, the accident of belonging to a loving and solicitous family who were deeply interested in me. I used to think that if I were poor and alone in the world I

139

should have been at peace, my personal life pared down to the slenderest dimensions, and the life of the imagination grown proportionately large and strong.

Those hours of writing had a shape, a fullness, and a solidity that ordinary hours did not have. They were round and full, like fruit. They were the fruit of each day. Without them the day was barren and sorrowful because it had no meaning. When those hours were rounded and complete each day, if I could have come out of an attic room where I lived alone and anonymous in some poor street in a strange city, I would have walked through the street with the ecstasy still hanging round me, I should have walked in a dream of bliss and goodness looking out upon the world and all its people with wonder and love. My own identity was like a chafing prison that I had escaped from during my magic hours, and even after the hours were gone each day my sense of being free still lingered. My heart went out to the whole world and I became one with it in a flood of joy and understanding. I had never been at home on the earth the way other people were, but now, it seemed, I had found a cure for my homelessness. At last I was at peace, too, like the others.

Alas! this happiness was only a magic spell and it could be broken in an instant, like most magic spells. Any of my family or friends could break it by speaking to me and making me answer them as the familiar Katharine they knew. In a second I could be thrust back into the painful narrow space of the identity that had been created for me by others. I was so young and my escape was so new to me that it seemed to me like a miracle, and whenever it was

140

annulled in this manner I felt a humiliation and a bereavement that I could hardly bear. My happiness seemed to me a very frail and vulnerable treasure. I had not learned then how strong it was. I had not learned how to lay it aside intact so that I could return to it again whenever I desired. I had not discovered that it is possible to move easily back and forth from one world into the other. Then, to me in my ignorance, each world seemed to eclipse the other fatally. When it was my own secret world that disappeared, for all I knew I had lost it forever. That fear almost made me die of grief.

The cruelest thing about the breaking of the spell in those early days was the fact that it was my mother, with her great tenderness and love for me, who broke it. She did it so gently, so unintentionally, it was a pitiful thing. She did it only by the way she treated me when I came out of my seclusion at the end of the morning. The humble searching solicitude in her blue eyes, her unconcealed pity and adoration fixed so intently on me, seemed to drag me back against my will into the body of the cherished invalid child. She had missed me while I was shut in my room, and she longed to have me talk to her and tell her what I had been thinking and writing. She could probably see in my face that I had been transported and refreshed in some strange happy realm, and she imagined that I could take her hand and lead her into it and let her see what I had been seeing. She wanted to share in every experience I had. Because I was so delicate and because I was deformed she believed that I would never leave her behind, even in my imagination, as normal children have to leave their mothers. I realized that she expected my poetry and stories to be the innocent roamings of the child she knew, the kind of work that anyone would expect from a talented, protected little invalid. But just as a very frail woman sometimes gives birth to a very strong child, I felt that I was carrying inside me something which had a robust life and a destiny of its own, unlimited by my physical limitations just as definitely as an unborn child's life and destiny are not limited by those of its mother. My work could be therefore, and was, a fierce contradiction of anything my mother could imagine that I would do. It was the work of a strong other self hidden inside me, a fast-maturing other self that was not even acquainted with the gentle, childish little invalid, not even politely aware of her. The new self seemed even to be trying to show that the little invalid was only made of papier mâché and had never really lived at all. I was completely absorbed in learning how to take care of this new thing working in me—not to shelter or protect it as the little invalid had been sheltered and protected, but to make it work hard, to exercise and train it and give it room to grow. In doing this I seemed to grow strong too. When my mother encountered me after my morning's solitude an eclipse had occurred. This new creative ruthless impersonal being had moved entirely across the cherished child's orbit, and made it disappear. These two could not exist inside the same body at the same time.

Therefore it was impossible at that moment for me to respond to my mother in the way she longed to have me respond. And because it was impossible her insistent yearning solicitude which would force me back into my cage destroyed my happiness, and filled me with a sense of loss and stupid helpless anger. I was too well brought up ever to say angry things to my mother. And as always when anger is not allowed to explode it flooded my interior in a heavy, unhappy, sullen silence, and nothing would come out of me except sad miserable monosyllables. As we sat together at lunch my mother would watch me with increasing compassion and disappointment in her eyes. She was not angry with me, only anxious and bewildered. All through our lunchtime she would try to divert and amuse me. She handled me so carefully that her attempt to help me was always indirect. She never exclaimed, "You seem very strange! What is the matter with you?" Instead, in the face of my stubborn twisted gloom, she would tell me little genre stories, episodes in the kitchen, or something she had read in the paper that morning. To my jangled nerves, keyed up by the morning's work to an unnatural pitch of sensitivity and criticalness, her little stories only added to my rage and irritation; yet in telling them she herself became in my eyes infinitely touching and lovable because of her willingness to appear stupid if only she could help me. I could see, even across the chasm of my own silence and estrangement, how much more admirable and whole and sweet she was than I. Half an hour before I had been exulting in my own strength and love, and now I felt weak and forlorn. She was so humble and feminine that she almost broke my heart, but all unconsciously she was forcing me to be something that I hated to be, she was making me hate myself, making me change into an ugly-tempered, unnatural and almost masculine child. She laid herself open to me, she offered me

143

all she was and all she could think of, straining to give me even more than she had. On her own ground she was not stupid. She had a classic, scholarly mind. Her intelligence was like crystal, without sediment. She used words with a clarity and precision which I have envied all my life. She was a Greek, a classicist, while I was a sloppy Romantic. And because she lacked the artist's intuitive knowledge and aggressiveness and originality, which somehow got planted in all her children, she admired us all too humbly. She exaggerated the importance of artistic talent and yet she did not understand the vagaries by which it sought its ends. I could not bear to see her display her own unconsciousness of her much rarer qualities of thinking and feeling or the pathetic misunderstanding by which she blocked my way. I felt like giving a great animal howl of woe and love and pity. But I could not speak, I could never explain to her what I was feeling about us both. Tired and discouraged at last, she would suddenly drop her effort, and say in quiet despair,

"You don't love me. I can't make you happy—it's no use. I don't understand you."

That sudden direct cry, which came so rarely from her and meant so much, loosened me and brought a gush of aching helpless words out of me.

"It isn't anything to do with not loving you," I cried. "I love you more than you can possibly understand. You've got to believe it or I shall die."

"But you are not happy with me, I can't seem to make you happy," she said very gravely.

"I don't want you to *make* me happy! I *am* happy. In myself! I am the happiest person in the world, at times."

"You don't seem so. I'm afraid I can't see it," she would reply from somewhere far away from me, suffering in a kind of human sadness and loneliness which I had never experienced and did not understand.

"It's something you can't see. Nobody can see it, but it is true. It is wonderful!"

"Why can't you tell me about it then, let me share it with you, if you love me so much?"

When she came to that unanswerable question I would fling myself at her and take her in my arms, struggling to tell her with my caresses what I could never explain in words. She submitted passively. She didn't like my kind of caresses. They were too violent and therefore untrustworthy. Such behavior as mine, first harshly shutting her away from me, and then ardently wooing her, appealing to her in desperation for her mercy and understanding, had no relation to her conception of love. Hers was the kind of love which seems to me a form of genius. It is so deep and continuous that it makes no unnecessary sound, nor gesture. Like many New Englanders and like the aristocratic Japanese, she regarded intense personal emotion as such a precious sacred thing that it must be kept locked and hidden inside the breast. If it was real and profound it was too overwhelming to be given a direct expression, and only a person who did not really feel it and did not know what it was could be so insensitive as to bring it to the surface voluntarily, or would profane it with the sensuous language of the body. Extreme understatement, entire lack of display, were to her the necessary guarantee of sincerity. Because I was inconsistent, changeable and violent in moments of

145

emotional stress, nothing I said or did at those times ever rang true to her, I realized. In my moments of worst despair she could never quite believe in me.

This scene was repeated at infrequent intervals several times during those years. Each time it happened it had the effect upon me of a heartbreaking surprise and disappointment. For in the interval between I fostered a necessary illusion in myself which was shattered each time this scene took place. It was more than an illusion, it was a belief I had to cling to, that my mother really, in her heart, understood everything about me. But even at the end of the scene, when we kissed and my mother sadly and skeptically said she would try to believe I loved her, nothing was settled. Nothing that either of us could say brought us any nearer to true understanding. But since her desire to give me whatever I wanted was stronger than her desire for her satisfaction she accepted my hours of seclusion, and she submitted in silence to the gradual vanishing of the dependent little daughter who had once been so sunny and companionable, the joy of her heart.

I ought not to tell such a story of hard and obstinate discipline and of the sadness I inflicted by it on my mother and on myself unless I could also say that in time I brought fame and happiness to us both. That is the proper way for such stories to end. But the point of this story is that there was no such brilliant reward for my pain and hers. There was no visible reward.

If I had had success my devotion would have been a very different matter. I would not have needed to be obstinate. I would have been praised and my working hours would have been eagerly and proudly protected. There would have been a genial feeling of elation and importance all round me. But year after year went by and I published almost nothing, and I earned no money, and in spite of it I continued to insist on my hours of work and solitude. I took my routine as seriously as if I had been Flaubert, who said, "I now lead a holy existence, I who was born with so many appetites. But sacred literature has become a part of my very being . . ." and of whom de Maupassant said, "He had given, from his youth onward, all his life to letters, and he never took it away. He used up his existence in this immoderate, exalted tenderness, passing feverish nights, like a lover trembling with ardor, falling from fatigue after hours of taxing and violent love, and beginning each morning from the time of his waking to give his thought to the well-beloved."

Sometimes it frightened me. It came over me with a wave almost of horror that after all I was not Flaubert, and that there must be something queer and crazy the matter with me which made me need this perpetual act of devotion so badly. When an interruption came and with it the intolerable malaise I was bewildered and heavy like someone torn out of sleep to whom being awake means painful suffering; and I would beat around stupidly in all directions trying to get relief. Then like a screaming baby who has been taken away from his mother's nipple for a minute in the midst of suckling and, without knowing what is the matter with him even while he kicks and screams, is hunting with a blind, furious, and true instinct for his mother's breast until he finds it again, so my instinct working through my blind stupidity would always get me back somehow or other to the infinite breast that was nourishing me, and I would be able to be still and spellbound again.

In accepting and indulging me in what must have seemed to her a joyless form of existence my mother was of course humoring me instead of understanding me. The feeling that I was continuously being humored rather than understood made me uneasy. It made me want to hurry fast and accomplish something that people could see. To be humored in this fashion is to be put under an obligation. It is like living year after year on advances from a hopeful publisher and never turning in a manuscript. I felt that in return for the child I had taken away from her I owed my mother some visible accomplishment that would somehow give me back to her in another form. As year after year passed and I failed to make restitution the sense of my debt became almost unbearable. Finally, because we could not live happily together, I evasively and guiltily parted from her and lived alone. But even when we were apart I continued to long for the luxury and the release of having my mother once fully understand me, instead of humoring me. I wanted her to understand and really believe that the reason why I refused to give myself to the demands of ordinary human life was not because I was selfish but because I was trying to give all of myself to one thing, to the absolute demand of art, which seemed to me very much the same thing as the absolute demand of God. But if ever I tried to explain this feeling I was clumsy and tongue-tied and apologetic before her, and the things I said sounded pretentious and unjustified.

But although I felt driven by the falseness of my situation, and as if I must, *must* hurry in order to

148

clarify it, something in me kept me from hurrying. I felt in myself a deep regular rhythm in which there was no such thing as haste. It was a rhythm of untroubled, imperturbable, profound, obstinate slowness—regular, exact, and deliberate, like a grandfather's clock. I felt intuitively that this was my tempo, the one that would bring me whatever experiences or rewards were destined for me. Even if it ate up years of my life before it brought me anything I knew simply that I must obey it.

If it brought at last some visible accomplishment, very good—if it never did I would not complain. It was the root of my life, and without the root there could be no flower. If I yielded to impatience, and to the hungry, human, youthful desire to be known and praised, and if therefore at times I rebelled passionately against that slow inner rhythm which kept me back, then I always felt guilty as if I were wronging something deep and mysterious that had been given into my keeping, and I turned back to my obedience. In allowing myself to be governed by this feeling year after year I had to resist very strong tempting things. In America there was a renaissance in progress, there was a new generation, and it was my own generation, of brilliant young people. I felt as if I were letting myself get left far behind. For to my dismay the talented, talked-of ones kept getting younger and younger. The *Dial Magazine* had been revived and was of great interest and importance to all the young writers and artists. Inside the front cover each month they printed the age and birthplace of each contributor beside his name. I always dreaded to look at that page because, though at first most of them were a little older than I, very soon they were my own age, and very soon after that they were younger, and when finally they began to be born in 1900 and 1905 it was lucky for my peace of mind that then the *Dial's* career ended, and I did not have to look painfully at that page any more.

However, it was impossible even after that for me to be unconscious of the fact that my contemporaries and others much younger were already making names for themselves in the arts. I followed their careers with minute eager attention. I read their literary reviews and articles and bought their works fresh off the press and read all the news about them wherever it appeared. Their books, their exhibitions, their names in print, news of their successes, their parties, marriages, divorces, their departures to Europe, their returnings to New York, excited me through and through. It was like hearing a rousing flare of band music a block away, and it was like being the only child in the block who, hearing it, stood still, while all the other children's feet went flying. For I had to resist not only the impatient longing to be known and praised for accomplishment, but also the furious, wistful longing to go where the others were in Paris or New York, to mingle with them, and to have the enticing modern experiences that they were having and writing about. But something in me kept telling me that it wasn't time for me to go yet. I had chosen what had to be, according to my conception and practice of it, the loneliest of arts, and sometimes I had to stop up my ears so that I should not hear the gaiety and excitement of the ones who evidently did not think it was a lonely art.

So I had reached the age of thirty-four, with all

my imaginary life and experience recorded in little heaps of unpublished manuscript, with no actual or worldly experience to my name and in an almost nunlike state of innocence. Nothing to show for myself at the age of thirty-four—"I who had been born with so many appetites!" It was a frightening thing. Yet I stubbornly refused to let time frighten me. I had got a harvest to reap from those years, even if it was an invisible one. I had learned to fasten my life to an abstract thing and in doing this I had learned devotion. I had learned to let impatience and despair slide off me—these few simple yet difficult things.

Now I had found my house, and the idea began to dawn on me that I could make it into a divine place where the writer's way of living would be the normal one. The understanding and protection of those special needs would be established as everyday necessities here in my house, in the midst of a delicious country life. I had read George Sand's letters to Flaubert written from Nohant where she was living with her son Maurice and her grandchildren, combining her hours of work with her sensitive enjoyment of country life, and with the pleasures which she and the children shared together, their games and marionette shows, their swimming and sailing. It was a life of strength and joy and accomplishment. The writer was mistress of the house and her work marched on. It was the central function of the house, taken for granted like eating meat and vegetables and drinking red wine. It was inconceivable that she should, like me, ever feel apologetic toward anyone for being a writer, or should ever have to explain and adapt her working habits in order to make them intelligible and acceptable to others. It was also inconceivable that she should ever need to use a childish defiance in order to protect her right to do her work and to be wholly and freely herself.

I wanted to create such calm security and happiness not only for myself. I was thinking too of other people unknown to me who were tormented by the same need and unable to satisfy it. I knew there must be many young lonely ones who were trying desperately to guard within themselves a small new fire of devotion to the search for truth and experience through the medium of writing; who did not know what was troubling them in their failure to do it, who lived in such alien surroundings that they had never heard that there were such people as themselves in the world, and who might decide perhaps, in failure, that it was not worth while for that fire to stay alive. I wished my house could be a refuge for such humble, anonymous, groping ones —not only a refuge, but a place of rebirth, a starting point for great destinations.

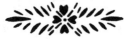

21

MY second wish was to make it an aunt's house. For when I had reached my quiet resigned thirties I liked aunthood the best of all the relationships that were open to me. Even Flaubert had a niece, and at the time when I bought my house I had two nephews and five nieces.

The Little Locksmith

Most children treated me as if I belonged to their world rather than to the grown-up world, and I was flattered by this great compliment. It was partly because of my small size. I had never grown any taller than a ten-year-old child and therefore children could never believe that I really was a grownup. At regular intervals my nieces and nephews would ask me again if I was ever going to grow any taller, if I was really and truly a grownup, and if I would ever be able to marry anybody. Ranie and Kitty and Ann, the three little sisters in a row who were my sister Lurana's children, were the ones who used to talk to me the most intimately about everything almost from the moment they were born. They were always wondering and talking most fantastically about such things as marrying and dying and God. They were not high-brow little girls. They all three quite lackadaisically took it for granted that they would become movie stars a little later on, but in spite of this frivolous aim they spent most of their own private time much less frivolously than most grownups do, in talking about the only things that are really important. When these three asked me questions about myself and the shape of my body they spoke of it with a kind of awe, as if they thought there was something wonderful about it—as if my difference made me more rare and precious than ordinary, properly made people. Yet in spite of this attitude they always spoke about it with a careful tenderness as if they were afraid they might hurt me; and whenever they talked about me and my deformity they would surround me and close in around me as if they wanted to protect me from something outside. For of course they had heard grown-up

153

people and other children of the kind who echo grown-up people's ideas speak of me in a very different way. They knew that the general grown-up idea was decidedly not that something rare and wonderful had happened to me. But children, if they are let alone, have their own strong and independent sense of values. They seem to value particularly anything which has escaped from the conventional pattern of grown-upness. And I had done this most conspicuously, although involuntarily. I always felt myself especially honored because the thing which seemed a misfortune in the grown-up world made me belong near the top in their independent, upside-down, antigrown-up scale of values.

The conversations between us concerning my deformity always occurred when we were alone, never before any parents or other grownups. Alas! If any of the parents had happened to come in during our conversations—my sister or my brothers—they would have been, like any other sensitive, well-bred people, horribly embarrassed. Because of the subject which had been so carefully repressed all of our lives they would not have been able to meet my glance without pain and confusion, if they had come in and found the children talking easily about it with me. The children's naturalness, graced with so much love and imagination and delicacy, was a wonderful and a new experience to me. They unlocked a lifelong barrier in me, and so they made me feel more at home and more at ease in their world than I had ever felt in the world of grownups, where this problem had been excluded from every conversation or, if by some awkward accident it did protrude above the surface, was met with dreadful embarrassment and a quick changing of the subject. This evasion was to me mysterious and terrible and baffling. I understood that my mother could never speak of it, and I understood that my brothers and my sister could not speak of it. And I understood that perhaps I could not have borne it if they had spoken of it when we were growing up. But the children, when they arrived on the scene, created a new dimension in which they and I could speak of it easily. For us it was so simple. I felt as if I had been a person in a fairy tale who had been locked up all my life in a lonely hut in a forest, and then one day children had come to play around my hut, and playing, they had found a key in the grass and just by chance they had tried the key in the door of the hut, and had unlocked the door and found me. They had gaily welcomed me and invited me to come out of my prison and play with them.

Earlier in my career I had had a critical experience which for a little while had threatened to make me feel that children were my worst enemies. When I made my first appearance in the perpendicular world, at sixteen or seventeen years of age, after spending most of my life in a secluded and horizontal situation, I began to walk out alone in the streets of our town for the first time; and I found then that whenever I had to pass three or four children together on the sidewalk, if I happened to be alone, they would shout at me, and call me by the terrible name which I had heard long ago describing the little locksmith. Sometimes they even ran after me, shouting and jeering. This was something I didn't know how to face, and it seemed as if I couldn't bear it. In the horizontal and protected place I had hitherto occupied inside the shelter of our home I had always been interested in younger children. My little sister Lury and her friends were always playing around my bed. I used to watch them and listen to their talk, and I never grew tired of their society. They posed for me while I drew pictures of them, and they were always asking me to make paper dolls for them, which I did for hours at a time. And between me and Fergus and Warren and their friends who came to play with us there never was any bad temper or quarreling that I can remember, and therefore I was completely unprepared for hostility from anyone, and especially from children, when I went out into the world, and least of all for those terrible and apparently automatic taunts and jeers.

For a while those encounters in the street filled me with a cold dread of all unknown children. My natural friends seemed to have become my natural enemies. I felt horribly exposed whenever I walked out of the house. And I got a sort of mariner's habit of scanning the horizon for my enemies and changing my course in plenty of time to avoid meeting them, especially the little idle groups of three or four which were always the most menacing. I could sometimes get safely past one child who was all alone. But no matter how cautious I was it was impossible to avoid meeting children. They would pop up out of a side street when I thought I was perfectly safe. They would suddenly come out of a yard or a front door.

This new danger contrasted strangely with all my past experience. It appeared that in the outside world I was seen very differently from the way I was seen at home. Among my family I was still the treasured, protected person of extraordinary importance, yet whenever I went out alone I was liable to become at any moment an object of contempt and mockery. Whenever the moment came and I had to walk past children, who were shouting at me, I used to try to seal myself up, get far inside myself, and close all my passages of communication so that their cries could not penetrate me and hurt me. For the reason why the children's cries could hurt me so was because I knew they were true. The children were perfectly right about me. They were the only people who were really honest with me. They made me share with them a horrible disgraceful secret concerning me which my family were too refined to understand. I felt that I had to protect my family from this secret disgrace of mine. If they ever should find out that I was being mocked at and humiliated on the street their horror would somehow make it even worse and more humiliating for me.

One day I suddenly realized that I had become so self-conscious and afraid of all strange children that, like animals, they knew I was afraid, so that even the mildest and most amiable of them were automatically prompted to derision by my own shrinking and dread. As soon as this dawned upon me I began to try to charm them like a lion trainer.

By main force I began to lift the focus of my own attention, and consequently theirs too, off myself and place it gently but firmly upon them instead. When they glanced up as I approached along the sidewalk they found me looking with interest into their own faces, as if I had noticed something quite astonishing and amusing in them. If they stared back without smiling I still managed to compel myself

157

to look into their faces invitingly while I still pretended to be unperturbed and lightly amused.

This method worked on them, and it worked on me. For I discovered that it was ridiculously easy to bend their soft and pliable attention back upon themselves, and then to make them unconsciously begin to feel a pleasant warmth being shed upon them, something even desirable and fascinating. At first it was only by a most desperate effort of imagination that I managed to summon up this ray of love and deep interest and direct it upon my enemies; but as soon as I saw that it worked my technique improved, and the charm worked better all the time until it suddenly merged into naturalness and was no longer a charm but the expression of real feeling. After that there was no fear or distrust left in me, and no child ever shouted at me again or, if any did, I didn't hear or know it.

After that, wherever I went, in subways or trains, or jolting through our county on the trolley cars of that period, I would always become fascinated by some child or other who was sitting near me. Often there would be a workman sitting opposite me wearing black greasy clothes and with a haggard tired face, and his wife, equally haggard and worn, and without a sign left on either of their faces of the freshness of their youth. And nestling between them there would be a child as beautiful as a little rose. The child would be tired and half asleep and dressed in poor cheap clothes, but its drooping dreaming face, its soft eyelids and heavy lashes and its miraculous fairness, its little chin and neck and voluptuous, unconscious hands falling over its father's or mother's shabby sleeve, could touch me with an overwhelming feeling of the beauty and pathos of life. Wherever I went, after this time, I always noticed them everywhere—children, who roused such feeling in me. I know that I used to stare at them in a kind of trance. They seemed to me the only beautiful human beings, scattered about like flowers in the midst of ugly, corrupted, grown people. They seemed to me like unearthly things, belonging to a world of perfection and innocence like William Blake's world. Unlike the race of grown-up people, children, it seemed to me, could never under any circumstances be ordinary or commonplace.

When I was young I could not bear to have anyone make life seem commonplace, and yet that was the thing that nearly all the middle-aged and old people did. I could not bear to hear droning middle-aged women tell about their stomachs and the gas that was or had been on their stomachs and about their constipated bowels. It was even worse when they talked about other subjects because they spoke of such things as childbirth and death in the same familiar and gossipy tone in which they talked about their stomachs and bowels. Such an absence of awe toward these miraculous things struck me when I was young as a horrible blasphemy against life. I could not endure it. I was shocked not only by their tone but by all the subjects which most of the old people spent their time thinking and worrying about—these subjects were not love and forgiveness and death and night and the stars, but sinks that had to be cleaned, the stock market, and that mysterious important monster whose name was Business, and whose health had to be inquired about and reported upon every day, as if he were a terrible old god whose good humor could make us all happy and whose bad days could plunge us into gloom. I despised the old people for allowing the mood of their immortal souls to be dependent on the whims of this monster. I said to myself that I would never submit to it.

I turned to children because they were free of all this corruption. They were the only ones who were not degraded by responsibility and practical calculations. They were the only ones who had any true naturalness, innocence, abandon.

Therefore when the new generation made its debut in our family, in the person of my elder brother's Tony with his wide-apart blue eyes and his little solemn questing spirit, I for one welcomed him with almost painful awe and tenderness. I felt that my new status of maiden aunt was the thing I had been waiting for, and the thing that would satisfy me. Of all human relationships aunthood seemed to be the one I was born for.

No, not born for. Nobody is really born to be a maiden aunt. In order to develop into a good maiden aunt I think you have to begin life like anybody else, born for a fine destiny full of hope and passion. Then you must have encountered some physical injury, heartbreak, or fatal misunderstanding which made it seem necessary to withdraw your hope and hide your passion and stand aside in the wings and watch the others who have been given real parts in the play.

These discarded people make the best, the only true and valuable maiden aunts. Their unspent love and the compensating talent, which they so often possess whether they develop it or not, can do certain things for children which no good mother ought to be able to do, since it happens that a good aunt makes a very bad mother, and a good mother could not possibly be a good mother if she had the wild erratic qualities which belong to the good maiden aunt.

Everybody knows that a good mother gives her children a feeling of trust and stability. She is their earth. She is the one they can count on for the things that matter most of all. She is their food and their bed and the extra blanket when it grows cold in the night; she is their warmth and their health and their shelter, she is the one they want to be near when they cry. She is the only person in the whole world or in a whole lifetime who can be these things to her children. There is no substitute for her. Somehow even her clothes feel different to her children's hands from anybody else's clothes. Only to touch her skirt or her collar or her sleeve makes a troubled child feel better. And often when a child wants her this is all that a mother has time to give. She is always moving. She has so many things to do. She can't sit down in a chair and talk nonsense right in the middle of a busy day. Sometimes a child has a great urge to talk what its mother calls nonsense. Sometimes even a child's worry about death and about the beginning and the end of the universe seems like nonsense to the busy mother when she knows by taking one quick animal sniff of him that there is nothing wrong with him.

This is where the good maiden aunt comes in. The aunt should have no binding domestic occupation. She should have nothing that could be called a domestic tie except the habit of being a carefree visitor in the houses where her nieces and nephews live. Or she may have the occupation of possessing a house of her own which is devoted primarily to receiving visits from her nephews and nieces and where there is somebody else to attend to all domestic matters.

The good maiden aunt is the one who is as free and nonsensical (and sad, at times) as the children are themselves, and who will never tire of paying attention to anything they may do or say. She is the one grown-up person in their acquaintance who will never look at a clock and tell them to hurry up because it is time for them to get ready. She would rather let them be two hours late to a dressmaker and three hours late to school than ever say this to them. Yet their mother could not possibly be like that, and the children could not bear it if she were. The good aunt has the same uncorrupted cosmic sense of leisure that the children have, and together they carry on conversations and enterprises which haven't any end. They lie on the floor and write and draw pictures. They make up songs, they make up games, they look at things through a microscope, they make things with scissors out of colored paper. There is no limit to what they may think of or invent. They discover wonders and talk about subjects that the mothers and fathers haven't any idea of.

The only occupation a good aunt may have apart from the children is something irregular; like being a painter or a story writer or an astronomer. Children can heartily sympathize with and approve of an aunt's doing this kind of work because they can see some sense in it themselves, and they can often be a great help to her in it. But even if the aunt never does any work seriously enough to become known in the outside world she must have come near enough to being an artist or an astronomer or a dancer to know how it feels to want to be one, or to want to belong to any other of the irregular, creative professions, so that she will recognize any such talent if it appears in her nephews or nieces. For some reason or other this kind of an aunt, especially if she never really does anything herself but remembers all her life the feeling of having wanted to, is almost sure to have at least one niece or nephew who shows signs of feeling the same thing. When this happens all the buried passion and unused strength of the lost artist in the aunt gathers itself up in her in one fierce purpose to help the unconscious waking artist or scholar or scientist in the child. The aunt can be very quiet about it, and nobody will know that she has this fierce purpose in her; but she will be continually on the watch and, without anybody noticing particularly, she will not miss many opportunities to supply whatever the child may need to keep the talent alive and growing in him.

The aunt will save her public fierceness for the moment of conflict which is bound to come—when the child grows older and announces his decision to his parents—his decision to be an artist, or a writer, astronomer, or dancer, or whatever it may be, instead of following the conventional career approved of by his parents. On that day the really good maiden aunt will show that she hasn't lived her inconspicuous frustrated life in vain. She will burst out in a great robust defiance of convention and in a championship of the artist which is quite equal in fierceness to the fabulous fierceness of the maternal instinct. I feel sure that behind many. of the great accomplishments in the arts and sciences which we have seen come forth in the world there was somewhere a now almost forgotten maiden aunt who furnished the extra ammunition needed for winning the decisive battle on some early day in an obscure, eager, young person's life.

But it isn't necessary to be the aunt of talented children in order to enjoy an aunt's life. That is simply one of the many possibilities. The good aunt always gives to any kind of nieces and nephews the something extra, the something unexpected, the something which comes from outside the limits of their habitual world. She is an aviator from another country who drops leaflets out of the sky. She does not intend to start a revolution, she only wants them to learn that there are other countries besides their own. She is the contradiction to the rhythm of their safe and cozy life which first awakens them so that their ears become aware of another rhythm, the rhythm of the unknown, the wandering and anarchical, the dangerous, the strange and wonderful rhythm of the world which exists outside of domesticity. She is the joker in the pack of cards which placed here or placed there can change the whole aspect of the game. She belongs to nobody and to everybody. She belongs now to one child, now to another, and the one whose turn it is to draw her wins.

This is the kind of aunt I rather hoped that I might be. I wanted to join the long line of the famous aunts of history: those individuals, sparkling and free, who left such treasures behind them—Jane Austen, Kate Greenaway, Louisa Alcott, Emily Dickinson, Robert Louis Stevenson's chief of our aunts—and Samuel Butler's Aunt Pontifex in *The Way of All Flesh*—aunts whose excellence in the role of aunthood is so richly shown in their lives and letters. Although my ambition was to be one of these maiden aunts of history I knew that I would be among the very last of the line. For it looks as if the virgin aunt would soon become an extinct type, since the withdrawal into spinsterhood after a heartbreak or in obedience to parents or, indeed, for any other reason, has become an archaic gesture.

Between the year of Tony's birth and the year when I found my house five other new members of our family had made their appearance on the earth. They were my brother Warren's and my sister's children. They were Jonathan Glover, Harriet Hathaway, and Elizabeth Keats; and there was my sister's exquisite little Ranie, and her Katharine, my namesake, who was the youngest newcomer at the time when I bought my house.

With this increasing number of nephews and nieces it was natural that I wanted to increase the scope of my aunthood. I wanted to put it in the right setting, on a grand scale. This called for a house of my own in the country. And so I dreamed my second wish for the life of my house, and it was a wish for the kind of eternal magic which a child sees and feels about a beloved place where he goes to visit in summer—a magic that will stay in his heart all his life long, and be a touchstone for all his life's experience—the place for which he is likely to feel this is a place that is not home, although it is as familiar and easy as home. It will have a strangeness and a wonder about it that home can never have. It is a place of poignant return and poignant farewell. It is a place enthralled, that waits and sleeps all winter long and is awakened again at the beginning of summer when the first eager footsteps go running over its threshold.

I wanted my house to be something of this kind, which would create a tradition in the lives and memories of the new generation.

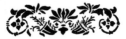

22

LOVE laughs at locksmiths. The adage had a twisted and a rueful meaning for me. I thought that Love laughed at me because my body was shaped like the locksmith's, but the answer I made was to unlock doors for everybody else while I myself remained a humble, submissive prisoner. My third wish for my house was that I might sometimes offer it for the use of lovers.

Having myself suffered from complete deprivation in this respect, I believed it was not right for anybody to be so deprived, and I wanted to do everything I could to prevent such suffering in other lives. I had not then learned that external circumstances are not the most potent causes of such deprivation. I did not learn until long afterward that a great part of my sense of imprisonment and consequent deprivation was caused by my own misunderstanding of the well-meant but harmful silence of my family concerning me. Many years later, when I broke the silence and reproached my mother for never talking to me when I was young as to how I was to deal with my predicament, she said that the famous Dr. Bradford who treated me had once spoken to her about the possibility of marriage for me, and he commanded her, "If she falls in love do not thwart her." When she innocently repeated that sentence to me, twenty years too late, I could not speak, I was so amazed. Then I said, "I wish I had known he told you that. I would have felt differently." She answered, ever so gently and remindingly, compassionately, "But you were not thwarted. There—there never was anybody—" I didn't say anything more. Inside I was crying, clamoring, "Oh, Mother! the reason why there never was anybody was because I was so afraid. You did thwart me! You did thwart me! by never talking to me and never encouraging me to talk to you! If I had only known he said that! If I had only known he didn't think it was impossible! You ought to have told me. You ought to have let me know. You have spoiled my life!"

When we were all young there was much gay talk and speculation concerning the current love affairs and the probably sentimental fate of my brothers and sister and their friends, but nobody ever said, "When Katharine gets married," or, "Why hasn't Kitty got a beau yet?" or, "We must get a beau for you, Kitty." I lived inside my cage, close to the others, among them, touching them, laughing and talking with them; yet by an unspoken understanding it was taken for granted that I was not to have what was apparently considered the most thrilling and important experience in grown-up life. Nobody ever put this feeling into words. Nobody explained the reason why. They didn't, of course. The reason was so obvious that no explanation was necessary. The reason was there in every mirror for me to see. But, given the reason, nobody ever attempted to console me, or to offer me any clue as to how I was to manage my life with this great thing missing. When I stood faced by an abnormal and peculiar difficulty my family who loved me and cherished me beyond any question gave me no help, no word. I used to think of going privately to see Dr. Bradford, to ask him what I was to think and do, but I could not endure the thought of presenting myself before anybody as an ignorant and pathetic person, and I did not go. I never was able to let anybody know that I was bewildered and afraid, and that a sneaking wistful hope kept springing up in a corner of my mind to tease and abash me, the hope that the Cinderella miracle might some day happen to me. In the dim background of that period I can now see my mother watching me and suffering for me, and hiding her suffering because she thought it might suggest painful thoughts to me that I had not yet had. She didn't realize that her silence harmed me more than anything she could have said.

Because I knew nothing at all about the psychology or the physiology of sex I never connected my deprivation and the silence which surrounded it with the almost intolerable malaise that I felt continually when I was young. I didn't know what was the matter with me. I only knew that my body never felt at rest, my mind never peaceful. I didn't feel at home in human life. I observed that there was a simple mindless ease and contentment which appeared to be the normal condition of other people. Things happened to them, they were worried and distressed by their difficulties, but they were always at home. They talked, worked, worried, did errands and planned meals, and everything they did came

168

natural to them as if, by an instinct I did not possess, they trusted and understood something that was behind it all. And when they were not worried or busy they could always sink at once into a pleasant relaxation of body and mind. They could listen to rain and be deliciously lulled. I would listen to the divine pouring of rain on a spring night and wonder, in silent terror, if nothing was ever going to soothe me, ever going to make me feel quiet and easy in the world. If the beautiful sound of the rain's lullaby could not lull me, and my soft bed and my family's love for me, I felt as if I must be incurable. I remember two particular times when something happened that made that feeling of despair cut into me so deep that it left a scar. The wound healed long ago, but the mark remains in my memory of those two things.

We went down the river in our canoe, my brother Warren and I, one afternoon in early spring, when the first thing happened. Canoeing was one of my brother's favorite recreations and he used to like to have me go with him. After he had paddled for a little while that day he drove the canoe against the soft bank and we got out and sat on the soft ground. It was the first warm day in April, the first time we had sat out of doors and smelled again the curious sharp smell of the spring earth and felt the sun so warm. I ought to have been able to enjoy it. I ought to have felt an immediate response to it in my bones and flesh and nerves and mind, the way every other human being in the world, I believed, except me could do. But even with the sweet sun on my face and with my fingers touching that fragrant earth I was still tormented. The powerful anesthetic of Nature could not work on me and make me forget my chronic malady. It only made it more painful than usual.

I sat up, stiff and shy, near my brother. I watched him. I could see how he was responding. To him the spring sun on his body was like a magnetic and beloved hand that had come back after being gone for a very long time away from him. He smiled lazily. He undid his collar, unbuttoned his shirt, and lolled at length on the moist ground. When he turned to look at me he blinked his eyelashes with a lazy, enjoying smile as the sun's humorous fingers played over his face. He was a happy animal, in harmony with the earth and at home there. His smile showed me that he was in the secret. Oh, why, why couldn't I be in the secret too? I could only watch him and sedulously pretend that I too felt at home. As usual I tried to conceal my despair. My queer suffering meant that I was an unitiated outsider in human life and it made me ashamed and I would have done anything I could to pretend not to be. I stretched out on the ground, pretending to be easy and relaxed, while I was perpetually wondering if I should ever in all my life find anything to do with the huge, tormenting, pushing load of passion that was in my chest.

My brother spoke to me, almost in a whisper.

"Look!" he said. I followed his glance. A big turtle was lying on the bank quite close to us, just beyond my brother. He was staring at it, and he motioned to me to move nearer so that I could see. I crept around close to the turtle, and stretched out on my stomach and leaned on my elbows. The turtle lay with her hind part at the edge of a smooth hole in the earth. She had dug the hole and shaped it to suit her purpose. It was a small opening like a tunnel that led down into a round shallow room below. A little heap of earth lay beside the hole. She had made her preparations and now she waited, utterly still. We waited, with our bodies still, scarcely breathing, and our eyes intent. Presently an egg dropped down the tunnel. Then we saw her stretch a hind foot slowly out and reach down into the little cave and place the egg just as she wished it to lie. There followed a long interval during which we all were still. With no haste, no motion, no struggle, with only a deep, deep stillness and tranquillity she waited. Then she dropped another egg into the earth. Again her skillful hind foot came out from under her shell and reached down and rolled the egg into place.

I envied the mother turtle. It was an envy that hurt me so much that I have never forgotten it. Unlike me, she was submitting mindlessly, in tremendous leisure, to the great tranquil scheme that contained her and governed her. I couldn't imagine any happiness to match it. We lay and watched her for perhaps two hours, until the last egg had fallen into the hole. Then we saw the knowing hind foot reach out and with delicate skill brush the loose earth back into the hole until it was all filled and covered over; and then we watched her pat the surface and make it all smooth and firm exactly as if nothing had happened there. When she had finished at last she drew her foot under her shell again and lay still. I thought that if I could feel ever, even for a few seconds, a satisfaction like hers, I could endure my life.

My brother watched and commented on the turtle's act with the objectivity of a naturalist. I knew that I did it all wrong. Other people did not relate to themselves the things they saw. The opposite happened—the things they saw carried them away from themselves. My brother's attention could move upon or away from himself flexibly and easily. He could throw himself on the ground and let his mind swing lazily while his senses responded in their fullness to his surroundings. The next moment, if his attention was caught elsewhere, his mind could suddenly be alert and focused on something altogether outside himself. All of my family, except me, possessed the instinct for learning, in books or outside of them, and they got a pleasure unknown to me in acquiring any sort of knowledge—in observing, collecting, comparing, discussing. I was a lost and idiot soul among them because I was mired in my own secret quicksand. I was apathetic and stupid where they were ardent, and I knew that here again I was missing one of the things which made them feel at home on the earth. I envied them their intellectual pleasure, yet I despised it at the same time, because it seemed to me as if their complacent objectivity were an excuse for ignoring deep intimate things, which became terrible when they were ignored. I wanted, though, to be like them because they seemed so much happier and more peaceful than I was. But I was very stupid and slow and I had not learned how to do as they did. Since my eyes were as keen as theirs, when I used them, I saw the turtle as vividly as my brother did, but because while my eyes rested on it, during that April afternoon, I made it carry on its back the entire load of what I was feeling during those hours—the accumulated emotion of all my uneasy days and nights—it became for me a symbol, impossible to forget.

The other thing that happened also happened on the river, one summer day. It was a companion piece. My brother took me down the river saying he had found something the day before, when he went down alone, that he wanted me to see. It was something fascinating that he thought I could write a story about, he said. He wouldn't tell me what it was. He guided the canoe down the river in the midst of the blazing sunny marshes and fields, among dragonflies and big arrowroot leaves, and into the shady woods below the fields. He stopped beside a grove of pine trees and we got out of the canoe. He led me up over the steep riverbank and we came into a place that was like a room. The branches of a giant pine tree made the ceiling. The smaller trees of the grove crowding round it made the walls. It was a spacious, dim, cool room with a red floor of pine needles. On one side we saw a fireplace built of field stones laid in a ring, recently blackened by fire, and a blackened kettle lying among charred sticks where the fire had been. On the other side we saw a low wide bed, made of pine boughs. We also saw two rain-draggled garments, one lying on the bed and the other hanging over one of the branches of the tree. They were fancy-dress costumes—the costumes of Pierrot and Columbine.

My brother and I stared into the deserted room. It was like something in a short story by Thomas Hardy. We imagined a boy and girl at a gay country dance in one of the near-by villages, in Boxford, Middletown, or Topsfield, the villages whose farms and woods and marshes lie on each side of the river. A boy and girl, suddenly in love at a dance, too enthralled to go home after the dance was over and take off their fancy dress and go back to the ordinary humdrum of existence, had had the beautiful simplicity and daring to follow an impulse that was like a poem and led them to do this extraordinary thing. They had lived together for a night and perhaps longer in a secret room of boughs beside the river. Then they had gone, leaving behind them the evidence that told their story as simply as the words of an old English ballad would have told the same kind of a story, in the same spirit, merry and bold. While we looked we talked about it as if it were a mysterious fragment of manuscript we had found, conjecturing as to how it should be completed, the lost parts filled in, by our literary imaginations. I responded to my brother's fascinating discovery as I knew he expected me to do, seizing with an artist's delight the problem he had presented to me. But inside myself I felt something quite different. This was not a ballad, nor an idyllic, balladlike story by Thomas Hardy or by me. It was real. That was what moved me. It had happened only the night before last, and it made all our literary fancies seem prim and ridiculous. Something wonderful and real had happened in that room, and I wished, with a heart full of rebellion and desire, that I had been that daring, joyous girl.

Those two scenes, the turtle laying her eggs and the deserted room, are like two full-page illustrations in color, illustrating the book of my youth. The text is gone, the words forgotten, but those two pictures on the river remain as vivid in my mind's eye as if I were holding the book in my hands. I can stare at them the same way I did when the book was new, and I can feel the same way I felt then—not only the detached literary thrill I was supposed to feel and had learned to assume on every occasion, but something which was much more alive and urgent then, something which struck into me, intimate and personal. Just like an imaginative child who stares at the colored illustrations in his storybook and recognizes in them with explicitness and certainty things he has seen nowhere else before but has known intimately in his most secret dreams, I stared, in a speechless, motionless trance of recognition, and I became the mother turtle busy with the act of creation, I became the boy and girl swept up on their amorous escapade. In these two marvelous scenes I could sense a huge governing force in action. All three of those other enviable ones were in league with a divine will, they were in the secret, and because they were yielding to that mystery and obeying it, they were all going forward in a rhythmic dance. I longed to be seized by that mysterious will, and be contained by it, too, and made obedient and humble to it. Watching them, I could hear and feel the great rhythm of life almost touching me too—almost but not quite. Through force of imagination and desire I could imagine myself taking part in that great dance, but I knew from the evidence of my family's silence and from the evidence of the mirror that I was inside a cage where I must stay all my life, and I could never, I thought, partake of those moments of deepest happiness which were designed for everyone to partake of. They were designed for me especially, I believed, because in those two scenes they called me with such unbearable sweetness. They called me the way the Pied Piper of Hamelin called the children, but I could not go. I

175

was the lame child who could not follow. So I stared at them without speaking.

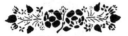

23

HAVING seen and surmised this much of what life held for those who could receive it, I angrily rejected the insipid substitutes which I saw other people taking up with who were not physically barred as I was, and which were offered to me. When my mother wanted me to settle down into a docile life at home, taking an interest in the meetings of the Danvers Historical Society and playing my mandolin in the Mandolin Club of the village ladies, and making little excursions on the trolley car to the Salem Athenaeum where I would sit, soberly and precociously reading the *Hibbert Journal* and Littell's *Living Age*, the prospect filled me with rage. I insisted on going away from home, I didn't know where. If I could not have intimate personal experience equal to the strength of my desire, then my instinct made me seek some kind of distraction which would be strong enough to equal it. This I found for the time being when my mother sent me to live in Boston, as a pupil in a boarding school which occupied a tall brownstone house overlooking the Public Garden. I loved novelty and the novelty of these surroundings enchanted me, and before I realized what had happened the load was gone. I became happy and eager as soon as I was there.

The city was full of a romantic feeling. I loved the rushing cataract of sound in the streets, of horses' feet and cabs and motor horns and policemen's whistles on a late winter afternoon, the sight of ladies and gentlemen stepping in and out of restaurants and theaters, the sense of movement and life, the surprises and the possibilities. I used to walk in the Public Garden and sit on a bench and watch the passers-by. For me, fresh from our country town, it was as exciting as the Rue de la Paix. Just to be there in the city, myself a part of the crowd, sharing with everyone else the brisk rhythm of the street, and that undercurrent of romantic expectant feeling in the air which made the city such a different place for me from the town of Danvers where the silence and emptiness of the streets was a deathly torpor. The city gave me the illusion for the first time in my life that I was mingling, participating. I used to look eagerly at one face after another in the quick-stepping throng on Boylston Street; I stopped to look at all the delightful things in the shop windows, and at the same time I learned carefully not to see my own reflection in those sheets of plate glass.

The atmosphere of the city also filled the interior of the brownstone house. I was happy in the school. The girls were mostly very simple-minded and kind-hearted and they did not intimidate me. With them as a not discouraging background, and under the eye of a gay, imaginative, sparkling headmistress who liked and admired me, I began to shine. I did not shine as a scholar, but I began just a little to shine as a potential artist and a social being. My forgotten childhood wit began to come bubbling out of

me again, and my talent for writing was taken so
seriously that I began to feel that I was fascinating
and important. At the end of my first year at the
school my English composition teacher, Lucia
Briggs, who was the daughter of President Briggs
of Radcliffe, otherwise famous as Dean of Harvard,
somehow or other made certain mysterious arrange-
ments so that I could be allowed to enter Radcliffe
as a special student taking the course in composition
given by Professor Charles Copeland.

I arrived at Radcliffe shy and countrified and
naïve from Danvers and my unfashionable school,
and yet from the moment when I first looked around
at the other girls I loftily scorned all the other shy,
dowdy, obscure girls like myself and picked out with
no hesitation the most interesting and distinguished-
looking young women in sight, whom I wished to
have for my friends. Lucia Briggs, on depositing me
at the Radcliffe gates, appointed Catharine Huntington as my senior, who would look after me, a fresh-
man. Catharine Huntington was one of those I had
already chosen for myself when I saw her standing
on a platform making a speech as head of some dramatic or literary society. She was beautiful and distinguished and talented. And even then when she
was so young she already showed the talent which
was to affect all the rest of my life so much, as well
as the lives of many other people. This was her talent to discern in an obscure person something rare
and important and to make other people see it too—
above all, to make the person in question feel it and
be it.

She could hold an utterly unprepossessing person
up in a certain light, like a collector showing a rare

178

piece, and the person, in her hands, would suddenly receive a value and importance which made the people who watched the transformation wonder how they could have been so blind as never to have seen it before. She worked the magic of transformation as I had never seen it worked before. She worked it upon places and upon experiences, upon everything that she saw or knew about. There was no coercion, no conscious, egotistical insistence in her attitude. She went about it just the way a gardener does, working by instinct, almost absent-mindedly, almost unconsciously, as he goes about among his plants through the day, turning one around an inch or two, setting another out of the wind, putting this one in a damp place, and that one in the full heat of the sun, with every motion removing from his protégés the disadvantages which continually threaten them, and which only he has the patience and the understanding to see and deal with. There are very few gardeners among human beings, and consequently most of the more difficult human plants are all in wrong places, suffering drought, or heat, or dampness, when if only a noticing, intuitive hand could move among them they might all flourish as they were meant to do.

Catharine Huntington was one of those rare persons, a gardener among human beings, and I began to feel a new warmth and charm shed upon me by her enhancing vision as soon as she was asked to look after me—just as if somebody had picked me up from a dank corner that had been all wrong for me and put me out in the sun. She disregarded, or didn't see at all, my delicate health or semi-invalidism. She spoke about my beauty, and I couldn't believe my ears. She admired my long thin hands. She treated me like a person who was rare and valuable and distinguished in some way. She treated me also as if I were a person of force, of exciting destiny out in the world, never for a moment like one who should be immured and kept inactive. She created and presented to me not only myself, a self that was new to me, but also a new world where people lived in a kind of Henry Jamesian atmosphere of thought and perception. She took me to stay at the old shabby country house in Lexington where she lived with her mother and two of her five brothers. I had no desire ever to go home again, and I accepted Mrs. Huntington's invitation to live there through the winter and go back and forth with Catharine to our classes in Cambridge.

It is not quite true to say that the atmosphere of the house was Henry Jamesian, because it was purely Huntingtonian, and it did not need any help from Henry James to be what it was. Sometimes in the evening Catharine would read Henry James aloud to me, but I was always more enchanted when instead of reading she would begin to tell me her own stories. Sitting on the edge of the harsh, narrow little bed she slept in, for she always disregarded physical comfort as of no importance, she would slowly brush her curling golden hair with a stiff English hairbrush while she told me about her five brothers and their lives, and about her friends and relatives in England, and especially about her favorite brother Constant, who lived in London and had given her the hairbrush from a London shop and her long string of real amber beads, and with whom she had lived for a year before coming to college. She told me about going to tea at Windsor, and at Eton, about visits in Amberley, and she told me how she had been given a party in London by Thackeray's daughter who was a friend of Constant. Little by little, when the story-telling mood came over her, she told me all of her great elaborate family history, about her aunts and her great-aunts, her grandfather the bishop, and her great-uncle Father Huntington, and about the old house in Hadley, and the beach cottage at Ogunquit. She would repeat to me some crucial conversation in her family of years and years ago, which had altered the course of lives. She told me about her young and wayward great-grandfather on her mother's side and the tragedy of his young Creole wife from Martinique, whom he didn't love and who was kept locked up by her mother-in-law in the attic of their old house in Salem. She told me about loves and hates, quarrels, estrangements, amazing marriages. And all the people in her stories had one distinguishing quality in common, which made them, either by blood or marriage, Huntingtons—a romantic race of people different from other people. As she told me her stories, she spoke in a minor key yet always with a kind of exquisite flourish and toss which showed me that although they, the Huntingtons, appeared to be required to endure more than the ordinary amount of personal tragedy, their spirit had never been defeated.

Even when she was narrating in her most sorrowful, minor key there was often a kind of unconscious playfulness and originality in her use of words, as there is when a child innocently uses language in a way of his own; and when this happened in the middle of a tragic story the effect was sometimes irresistibly funny, and I would burst out laughing. Instead of being offended and making me feel that I had ruined the sober splendor of her story, she would suddenly notice how funny she had been and she would laugh at herself, with peals of laughter. Her capacity for a shift of mood was one of the most amusing and charming of her qualities, and one of those quick breezes of humor did not alter the value of what had gone before. Everything about her was all of one piece. Still, her dominant mood was one of twilight melancholy, and she nearly always brought her nightly stories to an end with a Huntingtonian flourish, composed of a murmur and a sigh, and with her eyes downcast in sad meditation, she would shake her head slowly in the midst of its cloud of beautifully brushed hair, and fall into silence, forgetting me, and I would go wandering away to my own bedroom under the same kind of delicious spell as if I had just heard read aloud another chapter in the most fascinating novel I had ever found.

She and her brother Constant had both said they would never marry, and that she would go back eventually to London and live with him. None of the young men she met at the Cambridge and Boston dances ever compared with elegant, charming Constant in her eyes, and she wasn't in the least interested in talking or dancing with them. She often said that it was much more amusing to be with another girl, and this was not strange considering the kind of rare creatures who had strayed into Radcliffe at that moment from the outside world. Caroline Dudley, Eleanor Clement, Catharine herself, and a few others composed the small constellation of the elect at Radcliffe in my day, and they all had like Catharine a more or less cosmopolitan background which was exotic and sophisticated beyond anything I had ever known before.

But they were not the kind of haughty girls I loved to watch in theater audiences and restaurants and whose glance at me I later dreaded and feared. Although the Radcliffe cosmopolitans were at ease anywhere, and their clothes had the fragrance of Paris about them, they were potential artists and rebels and therefore in rebellion against any conventional career that might be expected of them by their families. They were also in mild rebellion against the immature social life of the college. They were like a small company of grown-up people shut up for a little while in the midst of adolescents. It always seemed as if they must have wandered in there by accident, in a moment of absent-mindedness, and would soon wander out again. Yet in spite of their vagueness and aloofness toward the mass of basketball-playing girls, jolly and handsome, who strode over the campus, these others were the only ones who shared with the Harvard professors in the Radcliffe classrooms a certain secret; for they shared a grown-up understanding of the real purpose of the college, its intellectual purpose. Because of this secret there existed between them and the professors a rapport which was not even dreamed of by the girls who had come to Radcliffe in order to be typical college girls. This little company of the elect represented in that little world a similar dissenting minority in the outside world; they represented the artists, the aesthetes, the elegant Bohemians.

183

And this strange thing happened. Not only Catharine Huntington but the others of that circle treated me as if there were something wonderful and rare about me. It was not simply that they perceived a person of talent hidden inside a misshapen body and inside a great shyness, but they amazed me by actually liking my appearance. They again praised my long thin hands and my face. They looked at me with the fresh unconventional eye of artists and they spoke about me to each other before me with the impersonal authority of artists—as if I were someone in whom everybody with any eyes at all would see the things to admire that they saw. They encouraged my passion for beautiful clothes, which I had always considered an incongruous passion that it would be best to keep under control. They amazed me, they took it for granted that I should think of myself as a romantic figure.

In spite of their feminine, romantic personalities and their love of clothes they did not seem in the least absorbed in the thought of men and of marriage, like the girls I had known in Danvers. Catharine Huntington frequently expressed her disbelief in marriage, and her dislike of the effect of marriage upon people. Caroline Dudley shocked the wholesome Radcliffe girls by using the word "mistress" lightly. Those cosmopolitans unconsciously put in their place for me, and indeed completely demolished as far as I was concerned, the Danvers girls whose wonderful silliness had made me feel so desolate and worthless. Here were girls with beautiful bodies and faces and a background of fashionable, sophisticated society, girls to whom almost any experience would seem to be open, and they talked all

the time about pictures and poems, about Yeats and
the Abbey Theater, and they laughed at marriage
and believed it was something to be avoided if
possible.

In that new exciting atmosphere I never suffered
any more from the horrible feeling that I was dying
of starvation—a suffering which had been distilled
to its pure essence by those two excursions down the
Ipswich River. I wrote poems which were published
in the Radcliffe literary magazine, and because of
the impression they made among my friends I in-
dulged in a lovely feeling of exaggerated self-impor-
tance and a swiftly mounting elation concerning
that mysterious thing, my future.

But at the end of three years I had to go back to
Danvers. I didn't wish to become one of the per-
ennial special students we all laughed at, those
dowdy, sad-looking, middle-aged, and elderly ladies
who seemed to be spending their otherwise empty
lives taking course after course at Radcliffe. When
my friends left I was ready to go. Catharine, being a
poor clergyman's daughter, had to earn her living
and she went to Connecticut to teach in a boarding
school. For Constant had married, after all, the beautiful Gladys Parrish, and Catharine, unrebelliously
because she believed in a nunlike life, prepared to
live the life of a kind melancholy daughter. Caroline
Dudley left Radcliffe in the middle of a year because
she was impatient to go to New York and do things.
Eleanor Clement, who had been like me a special
student, left Radcliffe because she too had more interesting things to do. She kept house for her father
in a most fascinating semi-Bohemian style; and since
a beautiful and striking poem of hers had been pub-

lished in the London *Nation* it seemed the moment for her to sit down at her writing table instead of taking courses at Radcliffe. Her talent being such a truly distinguished one, it seemed certain that she would write many more poems and stories and would make a fine name for herself. I also wanted to begin. I had written a poem which was published in *Atlantic Monthly,* and also a story called "In No Strange Land," which had brought me a letter of praise from Mr. Sedgwick, and which Professor Copeland had read to his class, saying, "I sniff a future for that young woman."

24

I WENT back to Danvers and sat down at my table with a block of paper and a pencil in front of me. But I had received too much praise. I had no idea of the patience and humility required of the kind of writer who sits down at his table every day. I did not know how to do it, and I suffered an agony of chagrin and frustration. Then a kind of cosmic loneliness began to descend on me every evening, and it became so queer that it was like a sickness. The horror that had darkened my childhood came back and closed in around my mind again, and it spread swiftly until it swamped me. My physical surroundings seemed unsubstantial to me. The only things that seemed real were the unthinkable mysteries of space and time, and all through the day and the night the thought of those two question marks would flash through my mind like bolts of lightning until they shriveled and destroyed everything around me that was near and human. I began to be afraid to go out of the house; soon I was afraid of seeing my friends, even my family. Just as in my childhood, I felt myself sinking in a hopeless quicksand of pure terror. My happiness and great hopes were gone, mired and ruined with me, and I knew I could not live without them. I thought I must be going crazy. I tried to bury myself in my bed. I refused to get up or speak or look at anybody, except my mother, who used to hold me in her arms. My mother engaged a nurse to take care of me, and our old crusty bachelor doctor came and sat in my room, helpless and silent, every day. I astonished myself by crying, even in front of our doctor, I who had always been so controlled and so fiercely unwilling to be pathetic and pitiable—I who had never cried even when I was alone, because of my mother's example of stoicism. My mother was all warm and tender toward me, and now she anxiously urged me and encouraged me to cry. She seemed to want me to let loose all my tears at last, as though she understood better than I did what was the matter with me and wanted me to cry my fill. But even in the midst of my tears she never said anything that gave me any idea of why she thought I was crying—she appeared to be in spite of her sympathy wholly baffled as to the cause of my grief, just as I was myself. And since crying didn't cure me a new doctor came from Boston to see me, and he leaned over my bed like a soothsayer and he said crucial words to me. He spoke to me like a general urging his men into action, he challenged me to be brave enough to disregard and so disarm the terrors which, if I let them frighten me, would eventually paralyze my body and my mind.

That doctor's military treatment resuscitated me, and under its power I got up trembling and pale and went to Atlantic City, as he had ordered, with my mother.

But for a long time, two years at least, the terror closed around me again at intervals, and the doctor's military treatment lost part of its effectiveness. I could never forget his challenge, and it prevented me from ever burying myself in my bed again; but his order to me that I was to ignore the inward fear and suffering, although it helped me, did not cure me. Sometimes when I was walking along a Salem street the sense of mysterious unearthly dread would suddenly take hold of me and bring panic and loneliness and a feeling of imminent, terrible disintegration. I felt as if, exposed there on the street, my face was going to fall apart in a wild scream of horror, and my body collapse from sheer fright on the sidewalk; and with this coming over me I knew I would be unable to speak to any acquaintance who might appear at that moment, with the normal easy smile and the terribly bright cheerful remarks that people usually made to each other on the street. I thought that even people who didn't know me would notice me and would be startled by the strange look that I felt must be on my face. They would think I was crazy, as indeed maybe I was. I felt cruelly exposed. I thought, They ought not to let me go out alone in such a condition. They ought to shelter me and keep me where nobody can see me in this piteous state. But the doctor had insisted that I must do just this,

I must go out in the street alone and risk the coming of this panic, and conquer it. I was willing and glad to obey anybody who spoke to me with such authority as he, and so I forced myself to go on walking even when I felt as if I were on the brink of hell, and sweat poured out of me and my mind was whirling in confusion.

Then one day I found somewhere, on a page I have since forgotten, three words which had greater power than even the doctor's words. When I began to feel the horror coming on, I said to myself, "God within me . . . God within me . . . God within me." While I was saying those three words I felt and I knew that I was no longer alone. All of a sudden, because of those three words, I could walk along the street without fear. Saying "God within me" brought me an inrush of quietness and sweetness, a feeling inside me of dignity and wholeness which was not me at all, but something greater than I was, against which the horrors were powerless. Just by saying, over and over and believing as I said it, "God within me, God within me," I could send entirely out of myself the quick-spreading toxic fear and the disintegration it created. Perhaps this was a symbolic experience by which I unconsciously found relief for my sexual starvation. Perhaps the miraculous sense of peace which I got from saying "God within me" was a trick of the unconscious, which substituted a religious ecstasy for an ecstasy of the body. If this is true it only means that both ecstasies have the same source, they are friends and they are both divine.

It was wonderful to recover self-possession in the midst of disintegration, but the ability to walk calmly

along a street in Salem was not enough to satisfy a
person with such fierce desires and ambitions as I
think I had then. The horrors attacked me at home,
not only on the street, and I could not spend my
whole time saying "God within me." God within me
was like a hand that took my hand and prevented me
from falling. But I had to do more than not fall
down. If I was going to live I must go somewhere.
I must proceed. And I discovered at that point another essential thing which showed me where to go.
I discovered one of the things I had known in my
childhood and had forgotten in my confusion. It was
that I had eyes, not only for crying or for staring in
blind fear, but for looking and seeing. I discovered
also that the visible world is inexhaustible. My eyes
need never starve. Most people know these things,
but I was always too stupid and slow to catch onto
them in the natural course of life as other people did.
I never learned any of the simplest things until I
needed them desperately. Therefore I looked upon
my discoveries as the miracles which they are.

Adolescence had lured me away from the healthy
instinct of childhood which had known how to balance the unearthly, unbearable ideas of night by
the sane, humorous, and earthy little writings and
drawings of the daytime. With adolescence, I tossed
all that earthiness and humor away in scorn. Later,
my experiences with Warren and with my friends at
Radcliffe gave me an intense, romantic feeling about
myself, and filled me with vague and most disturbing desires which I expressed in intensely emotional
and mystical poems and tales. It was, indeed, the
almost unbearable unearthliness in what I was writing then which seemed to convince people that I had

an interesting gift. Then that unearthliness, so lacking in any earthly balance of real experience, began to frighten me as it had done in my childhood. It got beyond my control and then came the uninterrupted terror and the breakdown. And when I was all but lost in the quicksand it was once more the healthy instinct which rescued me and made me suddenly notice the objective world, and then come back to its healing powers again, and abandon forever my unearthly, mystical kind of writing.

After I had discovered my eyes I taught myself to remember them whenever the horrors struck me. No matter what might be happening to me, no matter how crazy and frightened I might feel, there was always the great visible world before me, and I could look at it. When a moment of terror came I could look at a chair, or at a table, or at a door, and by deliberately and faithfully looking at it and really seeing it with my whole attention, with the intense and humble and selfless concentration of an artist, of a child, of a van Gogh, I could realize and see the chair, or the table, or whatever the object happened to be that was in front of me, as I had never realized and seen it before; and it became for me in that moment an object of love, full of mystery and meaning, because the entire visible world became, when I really looked at it, lovable, mysterious, and significant. An ecstasy filled my hand and I began to work. And so I found out where I was to go. For by setting myself to work with the aim of translating my wonderful delight and realization of things into words and sentences I could deliberately cultivate the delight and prolong its visitations until it became the element within which I lived, safe at last, happy and

191

invulnerable. With my eyes and my hand I could save myself, by the grace of God, every time the powers of Evil attacked me inside the darkness of my head.

Even in the midst of my sickness, when I had believed I never would write again, the healthy instinct began to work when one day I had reached over from my bed to get a pencil and paper out of the drawer of the night table beside me and I wrote down on a little block of pink paper an idea for a novel that had fallen like a seed into my mind from listening to my nurse tell the story of her life. As soon as I had come home from Atlantic City and had discovered what my salvation was going to be I went and found my little memorandum on a pink slip of paper in the table drawer. There it was, waiting for me. It filled me with excitement and anticipation. It happened that for me and my purpose it was a living seed. Out of it a story grew and kept on growing year after year, curving like a vine first in one direction and then in another, yet creating and maintaining by means of its own mysterious will its own equilibrium and design. It grew as knowingly as a beautiful and intricate shell forms itself, or is formed by its soft, amorphous, yet accurately guided inhabitant. It was mysterious and beautiful to me, not necessarily to anybody else. But that was enough. I was in love with it, spellbound. It was a story about two sisters who lived in an old yellow farmhouse on the edge of Danvers. I watched every fly that crawled over the kitchen table in that imagined farmhouse, and I smelled every cake and loaf of bread the sisters made, and I heard the stamping footsteps of their father coming in from the snow.

I knew how they all felt toward each other, how each one thought and moved and worked and lay tired and alone in bed and fell asleep and woke again. I knew what the younger sister was thinking the night she ran away, and how the older one felt when she found the empty bed. By keeping my whole heart bent upon their hearts and my mind's eye faithfully and eagerly fixed on them—watching not merely their figures moving to and fro, but also their rooms and their dooryard and their neighbors' houses and everything else they saw—I was able to build up for myself what appeared to be an invulnerable calmness and joy, and a complete indifference to my own personal life except that it should remain empty and leave me free to live wholly in this new element which was not the real world but a kind of mirror element in which the essence and movement of the real world was reflected, as in a fortune-teller's crystal. It was then that I made Flaubert my model of devotion and began to learn the need for being humble. It was then that I discovered that I could make my life whole and peaceful by learning to be obedient to a power outside myself. And the more I surrendered my life in obedience to that power, the more I distrusted obedience to other persons who might have managed my life, and who often wished and tried to. "Un labeur courageux muni d'humble constance Resiste à tous assauts par douce pacience."

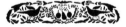

25

WHEN I began to live this dedicated life I was about twenty-five. After I had been living it for two or three years I began to feel as if I were a person who was living in the thick of intimate human experience. Thanks to the mysterious power being lent to me which made my imaginary experiences so vivid and satisfying, I thought I actually knew as much and perhaps even more than other people did who merely had full and eventful lives of their own. They only had one life apiece while I was living the lives of dozens. Because I believed it myself I began to give the impression to certain of my friends (who must have been a little lacking in real discernment) that I was very knowing and wise concerning the human heart, and they began to confide in me about their love affairs and ask me for advice.

It was almost as if my so-called nervous breakdown had been the equivalent of a tragic love affair which had made me superior and immune to any more of that kind of suffering. Actually it had not been the equivalent but it had had a similar effect. It had been an experience which might however be described as Thornton Wilder described love in words which I do not think can be improved upon, "as a cruel malady through which the elect are required to pass in their late youth, and from which they emerge, pale and wrung, but ready for the business of living." In the same way, my illness, or its cure, or both, seemed to have inoculated me against the desire for romantic love and made me able to view it in others compassionately and without envy. I had almost gone mad from loneliness, I had almost died of it, without anybody knowing and without myself knowing until long afterward what was the matter with me. I didn't understand what had happened. I only knew that I had not gone mad, I had not died of it. A block of paper and a pencil had saved me. They had not only saved me by satisfying my hunger and canceling the overwhelming terror of the universe, but they gave me also an inexhaustible form of entertainment because they gave me, or seemed to give me, the equivalent of all sorts of human experience. There was no end and no limit to this kind of living. Among all the people whom I knew I felt that I was the enviable one. I had substituted the invulnerable passion of art for vulnerable human passion. My circumstances were such that I was free to give myself wholly to the thing I had chosen, and I knew enough to know that such freedom is a very rare luxury.

I grieved to see my gifted friends, one after another, voluntarily letting their beautiful gifts go to waste because each of them sooner or later fell into the sickness of romantic love. I lost faith in women artists because I could see that for every one of them writing or painting was not a genuine passion, but only a temporary substitute or pastime which she was eager to lay aside instantly for the sake of a love affair or a marriage. I grieved equally when I saw nontalented human beings fail to live fully as human beings. I could not bear to see any halfhearted devotion in either direction, either to art or to living. At that unenlightened period in history the world was still full of a generation of devouring mothers who prevented their daughters' escape by all kinds of refined and sadistic obstructions, from weak

195

hearts and lonely widowhood to the simple, forceful ascendancy of the parent over the child. The great war between mothers and daughters was then only just beginning, and I was one of its most passionate fighters on the side of the captives. My friends probably thought of me as being much wiser than I really was partly because I was a separate person, looking on and meditating and partly because, as a partisan of the wistful daughters, I was always reiterating my belief that every human being must fulfill his or her own destiny. It must have been for these two reasons that my friends who were hesitating on the brink of perilous love affairs always confided in me and asked for my advice. They knew that I would be sure to give them the advice they wanted—that which was contrary to the world's and to their New England consciences. They knew I would urge them to go ahead and risk everything.

I did urge them. For my conception of love was that it was merely another form of man's assertion, which he makes in every work of art, that life is not ordinary. I was a fanatic in my belief that life is not ordinary, and in my hatred for all the acts, manners, talk, and jokes which treat the mystery of life as if it were comic and obscene, to be handled with contempt and laughed at or kicked around like an old rag. I believed that the experience of being born, of living, and of dying was all a poem, and that it should be received—all of it, every part of it—with wonder and gratitude. I thought that love was a power, like the artist's, which suddenly gave to a man and a woman together the sense of wonder. When I saw a man and a woman in love regarding each other with an intense awareness of each other's mystery and preciousness I believed that those two had for the time being cast off the corruption of ordinariness which makes most people blind to the miracle of existence. I believed that their sudden vision was like a saint's or an artist's vision. And I knew that when two unextraordinary people are in this state their happiness is in great danger. It is new to them and they do not know how to hide it and protect it from its enemies, and therefore it is in grave peril at the hands of those traditional enemies of the ones who see visions, those members of society who make and enforce the rules which are hostile to anything they themselves cannot understand, and who take upon themselves the right to treat the most sacred experiences in the manner of the police court. Whenever I heard or read in the newspapers about some poor devil of a hard-working respectable bank clerk or businessman whose career was suddenly ruined by the astounding discovery that he was keeping a mistress, I always used to imagine that he was a man who was merely trying to find for himself some reassurance that life is not ordinary—some escape from an existence that had been made intolerably unmiraculous for him by a prosaic wife. Most lives, I thought, lacking art, lacking religion, were choked and suffocated by the continual insistence of the personal, and of all its wearying insistent paraphernalia. I thought that husbands whose lives were so choked and suffocated with too much boredom and talk and anxiety and struggle wanted only a chance to worship love in the abstract, as it could be represented for them by an unknown woman or an anonymous girl in the darkness of an unfamiliar room. For this reason I believed

197

that even prostitution should be regarded not as something evil, but as a sacred ritual, as necessary for human beings as books and music and paintings are. I felt that my old favorite magic of transformation could show that it can be a good service just as easily as it can be a profane one.

And while I sat on my doorstep in Castine that first autumn I began to dream of a house as calm and still and beautiful as a work of art, where love might find refuge. Sex was evil, I thought, only where dignity or taste or any sense of holiness were not put into it, and when the wrong people for the wrong reasons have taken it upon themselves to satisfy one of the deepest of human needs. I began to create in my imagination a house restrained and severe in design, with no decoration except fresh flowers and perhaps some beautiful shells laid along a mantelpiece, perhaps a statue and a fountain. There would be, for servants, a staff of quiet, oldish women, brisk and clean and rosy, in white aprons, to carry meals and to wash the linen and lay it in herb-scented closets, and to keep every part of the house polished and beautiful. On the upper floors there would be rooms as quiet and remote from the world as a cave beside the sea, windows with stars in them at night and with inner shutters arranged in such a way that darkness could be summoned at any hour. There would be no sense of furtiveness and guilt in the darkness of those rooms; it would be benign and mysterious as the darkness of night out of doors; it would be like an ocean of forgetfulness fathoms deep, into which tortured unhappy modern man could plunge, leaving on the surface behind him the weary garment of his identity and all the

198

claims of the outside world that clung to his identity like pieces of lead. He would be light and free, and he would plunge deep into the darkness. The darkness in those rooms would be like a mighty bath of absolution and of forgiveness to the world for all its injury to his nerves and mind. The young women who chose to serve in my imagined house would be as wisely trained in the art of pleasing as Oriental women are, and would understand when to be still and submissive, when to be playful, when to be tender, when to lose themselves. They would have, if possible, the attributes described by Alain-Fournier as being essential ones, "audacious initiative and superhuman tact," and would be educated, as women, so it seemed to me who had had no such education, in the highest sense of the word.

A house such as I was dreaming of would be only another example, I thought, of the easy magic of transformation by which one thing becomes its opposite. All that was needed, I thought, was a person bold and independent enough to undertake it. That person would need to be very bold indeed, because the process of transformation was so entirely a matter of faith and magic and simplicity that nobody would believe that it could be done until after it had been done. I thought for several reasons that I might be the bold person.

Sometimes a worm will sew a stitch in a young leaf, and even though the leaf may partly unfold, and partly grow and live, it will always be a crumpled and imperfect leaf. My body, like the leaf, represented that mysterious element of imperfection in Nature, which allows the worm to maim the leaf; I represented the flaw which exists side by side with a design which appears to be flawless. Because the worm had sewed a stitch in me and made me forever crumpled, I belonged to the fantastic company of the queer, the maimed, the unfit. It was understood that I could not play a part in the ordained dance of love, in obedience to the design. I was obliged, therefore, in a certain sense, to skip in my own life all the years and all the force and strength which other women gave to love and to the bearing of children. I was obliged to skip the years of sexual activity and become, while I was still young and joyous, the equivalent of an old woman, a detached, sexless, meditative observer. But I was too sympathetic and ardent to be a passive observer. I had to act in some way. I had to participate, myself, in the ritual of love and experience. With my belief in the magic of transformation and my belief in my own power to exert it, I suddenly knew that I was the suitable bold person, the little, old, young crumpled person who could accomplish, if anyone could, this amazing project. I saw myself as the potent little figure, not old and not young, conspicuously lacking in size and in beauty, who appears and reappears in all folk tales as the good godmother, the talisman-giver, the magic-bringer, who inevitably comes to the rescue of young people who are much bigger and more beautiful than she is, yet who get themselves entangled in their life-size and more than life-size human troubles and are weak and helpless until that familiar little nonhuman figure arrives on the scene. I knew that my destiny would reach its mark if I could work this unheard-of transformation and make my house the place of refuge and solace I had been dreaming of.

I sat on my doorstep in Castine in the still autumn sunlight, and I began to be quite astonished and a little appalled by the things that I found myself thinking. But I did not let that scare me. For my third wish I wrote in my imagination across the panel under the mantelpiece in the square room behind me the last two lines of Shelley's *Epipsychidion.* "Come, leave the crowd which errs and which reproves, And come and be my guest, for I am Love's." I wrote them only in my imagination, but in my imagination they were always there, as long as the house belonged to me—the invitation which I wanted to give to all the people in the world who needed it. I might have written beside it, "Unto the pure all things are pure; but unto them that are defiled and unbelieving is nothing pure"; but it seemed to me it came to the same thing.

I wanted my house, then, to be a safe refuge for three kinds of people, who are all alike in being at a particular disadvantage in the outside world because they all possess and are guided by the mystic's innocence toward life, the fearless innocence which is not afraid of facing everything, and, facing everything, dares to believe, as Blake says, that all that is, is holy. My feeling of affinity toward that fundamental kind of innocence was the basis of each of my three wishes concerning the future of the house. It was the essential attitude which I wanted my house to prove possible and to defend.

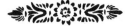

I SAT on my doorstep and admired the crickets in lazy joy, while I steeped myself in the sweetness and promise of my great possession and of my three great wishes. For the first time in my life I was able to sit at ease without needing the anesthetic of paper and pencil. I could do nothing and stare lovingly around me and feel a luxurious happiness, that simple gift which I had envied so much in others. My house and land were a token payment, which had given me kinship with the earth at last. Now even I was in the secret, rapturously at home. I remember how different my face began to feel, on account of a most unfamiliar sensation which came over it. It was a smile that simply couldn't leave my face for any length of time, and, constantly returning, it kept warming me all through. And while I smiled on the doorstep I could hear the workmen laughing inside the house. I could hear their footsteps and the slow rumble of their talk, and every now and then a great burst of laughter. Sometimes a fit of noisy hammering or sawing would discreetly drown from my ears the story or the joke that came just before their loud guffaws. Once in a while one of the men would come to speak to me about the work and ask me to decide something. They smiled good-naturedly, they were deferential toward me, and also protective, as they might have been toward a pleasant, well-bred child who for some reason had temporary authority over them. Their deference as well as their protectiveness seemed natural to me, because I think I felt that I was something set apart, a special and a rather important little package, containing ideas and talents and a vision of life which they were not capable of understanding. I felt toward them all, even toward Frank Grindle, who was different from the others, a rather prim, virginal, modestly superior, benevolent affection. As a workman and artist myself in my own medium, I had a fellow feeling toward them because of their workmanship, and I enjoyed the warm human reassurance I got from having them around me. What they thought of me I cannot imagine, but if they could have known the thoughts and plans that were in my head concerning my house, and especially the third wish, I suppose that not all their hammers and saws going at once in full chorus could have drowned their wild peals of laughter. With all of my alleged advantages, sensitiveness, talents, reading, friends, cultivated family, sweet temper, philosophical calmness, conquest of despair, and altogether refined superiority, I had still quite a long rough road ahead of me before I should have learned as much as the laughing workmen knew.

At first when the men and I had been talking over the work and I had described what I wanted done, or later on, when I had watched and commented and made suggestions as the work developed, the men had all told me at one time or another how smart, or bright they thought I was. They said it in a very friendly, beaming way, as though they really admired my brightness and took real pleasure in praising me. In paying me their compliments they seemed even rather possessive and proud of me, a little as though I were a child they had adopted. I discovered later that they be-

lieved, like my nieces, that I was not really grown
up. For when my birthday came on October second,
and I was thirty-four, Lorna and I talked about ages
and we found that we were the same age. She declared she couldn't believe I was so old. She thought
I was ten years younger than herself. Then she told
me that when I first bought the house people in the
village were talking about me, and reported that I
was a young girl of seventeen; they were all saying
how strange it was that I should be allowed by my
family (if I had a family, which some of them
doubted) to buy a house all alone. When Lorna told
me this quaint piece of gossip I laughed, but she
said emphatically and quite seriously, "Don't tell
anybody your age. Let them go right on thinking
you are a *very bright child!*" I found it so charming
that I quietly followed Lorna's advice and kept
right on, as long as I was able to manage it fairly
easily, being a very bright child.

I was used to having some casual acquaintance
mistake me now and then for ten or so years younger
than I was, but I had never met anyone before who
had taken off quite so many years from my age as
the Castine people. My nurserylike hygiene, which
my mother had impressed upon me as being necessary for my health, may have preserved a certain
freshness in my appearance, but whenever I heard
anyone express surprise on being told my age it
made me think of Alexander Pope, for one of his
contemporaries had said something about him that
was equally true of me. "His body," he said, "is
shaped like a pair of scissors, and he has the face of
a child." Then another contemporary, on hearing
the remark, added, "Yes, but it is the face of a child

who has been in hell." I felt curiously guilty when nobody made that amendment in describing me, for it seemed to me that somewhere in my young-looking face, and, if nowhere else, surely in my eyes, must be the evidence that I was another such experienced child. I had been initiated into an awareness of things that my parents did not even dream of, and I still carried all by myself a constant awareness of the fatal principle of imperfection, of accident, of mutilation, and of obstruction which exists in the universe side by side with a design that appears to be as flawless and symmetrical as a snow crystal. Instead of feeling pleased and triumphant when anybody said I looked very young it almost always cast a shadow over me, a somber uncomfortable feeling as if I were carrying a dreadful secret that was being concealed from them. I did not feel this way about the mistake the Castine workmen made, for I thought I was much more mature than they and I had become so through my prolonged suffering and inner life of imagination. It was going to take some little time for the education by Castine to break through, some little time for me to learn after all that I was exactly what the men had thought me—nothing more than a very bright child, too bright, so bright I hadn't even known enough to grow up.

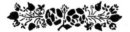

27

PRESENTLY, as winter approached, it grew too cold for me to sit outside on the doorstep and too cold for the men to work any longer inside the house.

During the long Indian summer while I had been sitting on the doorstep, building something in my imagination which I innocently believed was the future of my house, the workmen, by their loud, enthusiastic hammering and sawing, had accomplished things which I found very refreshing to my senses each time I aroused myself from my thoughts and abstractions and walked into the house and I could see and touch what the men had done, and we could talk about it together. I could smell the dramatic smell of new plaster and new wood in the midst of the autumn smell of Castine. When the cold weather came and stopped their work Mr. Gardner, the mason, had finished building the brick fireplace in the west sitting room in the same spot where the original one had been taken out, and Mr. Dek Littlefield, the carpenter, had put back the carved mantelpiece which used to be over it. The former owner had long ago removed this mantelpiece, finding it distasteful, as well as another from one of the bedrooms; but by some strange good sense, instead of breaking them up and putting them in the kitchen stove he had laid them carefully down on the attic floor and saved them for the last fifteen years, probably in the shrewd hope that if he waited long enough he would surely encounter a buyer just as foolish about such things as I had turned out to be.

In the act of putting things back in their places in

206

my house I found an intense curious pleasure, especially in the room where the carved mantelpiece went, because there it did so much. There it seemed like an act of grace. As soon as the mantelpiece came back where it belonged, a certain feeling seemed to flow back into the room. It became a cherished place. It became gentle and alive.

This was, evidently, the best room. It had a wainscot all around its walls, made of one board so wide that the men said it must have been cut from some huge primeval tree at the time the house was built, in the year 1800. Along the top of the wainscot an unknown hand had carved the rope design. The same rope motive ran along the cornice at the top of the room, and it was also carved on the mantelpiece. So, when the mantelpiece was put back it completed the unity and design which had been intended in the beginning.

The architectural adornment of my house was very simple. It was not especially impressive compared with the elaborate carvings I was used to seeing in the famous Salem houses. But this shy country elegance in a house which stood alone among hayfields on a Maine peninsula appealed to me. Because of its remoteness and simplicity this elegance seemed to me even more worth admiring than the richer elegance of the famous houses. Part of my pleasure in taking possession of such a house was the sweet triumph of saving something whose creation in that remote village must have been almost a spiritual achievement, and of seeing it emerge and live again, unperturbed by the previous owner's ignorance which had come so near to obliterating it entirely. This was a great chance for me to try to work the

207

so easy and so little-used magic of transformation.

The first thing I tried to do that autumn was to obliterate in their turn most of the crimes the previous owner had committed. I had the men soak off his terrible wallpapers, and pull out his terrible chandeliers. But there was one of his crimes which I allowed to remain. It was a large plate-glass window which he had let into one side of the room where the rope carving was. I meant to change it later, but after I began to live in the house I discovered that, although it was architecturally a sin, I used to love to lean at that window and find myself almost out of doors, looking down at the deep-blue-green grass tumbling around the trunks of the apple trees. In late spring when the two old apple trees were covered with their white bloom they seemed to come right into the house, through the big window. So I grew fond of it and let it stay. That graceful room, full of sunshine, on the southwest corner, was the room destined to become the one most used and most loved of the entire house. Wonderful, strange things happened to me and were said to me there, which I never could have believed were possible at the time when I was so eagerly preparing it. When I look back at myself, I appear to be wrapped in the earnest innocence which almost every person appears to be wrapped in if you can sometimes look back upon him from a later period which was then to him the unknown future. Because I know now what was going to happen to me, my past self looks incredibly naïve and unconscious, going about her preparations.

And now to go back to what I was doing then so earnestly. We had accomplished before the cold weather came several other interesting things besides the fireplace and the mantelpiece. Mr. Littlefield had moved the cellar stairs from underneath the front hall to underneath the kitchen, so that where the cellar stairs landing had been we made a most convenient little retiring room, with a washbowl, electric light and mirror, tucked in neatly under the slanting ceiling made by the front stairs. I was still not supposed to climb stairs any oftener than necessary, and I felt pleased by the easy adaptability of my large romantic house to my physical limitations. I relished the working out of these practical details. I tried to work them out with the neat precision of a good game of solitaire, and I got just the same kind of fun and excitement from it as from playing a magnified game of solitaire and making it come out.

After we had finished the successful little creation under the front stairs we made a new landing for the cellar stairs out of an extra kitchen closet, with a place at one side for mops and brooms. Next I bought new twelve-paned windows for the entire house, for my predecessor had removed the original old twelve-paned ones and had put in the three-paned kind. As everyone knows who ever looks at houses, there is something inexplicable about those three-paned windows, in that they can make any house look as if the life going on inside it were a life of unspeakable boredom and dreariness and despair. Change them for twelve-paned windows and immediately your house becomes cheerful and enticing, relieved of that strange pall. Yet all over New England, when the large-paned windows were introduced, indulgent husbands bought them to please their wives because they were so much easier to wash, and the charming many-paned windows were discarded. Even at the late date when I arrived in Castine somebody was as happy and proud to get the windows I discarded as I was to be rid of them, and I sold them all for nearly as much as I paid for the new ones. I was much pleased with myself for this sign of the business acumen which was so highly valued in my family and toward which I had always felt rebellious and scornful. I found it was exciting, like having my game of solitaire come out again.

I made still another exchange with my predecessor in which both of us exulted because each believed the other was a fool to be so glad to get a worthless object. I got back the old front door of my house which he had taken out and replaced with a fancy golden oak door from Sears and Roebuck. He thought the original door was not fine enough for his residence, and he put it into his place of business. When I asked him to exchange back again with me he did it with alacrity and teasing triumph. The thing I liked best about the old original door was the way its panels, set with narrow, handmade moldings, made a great serene sign of the cross—two short panels at the top and two tall ones below. It was a beautifully proportioned cross, ample and calm, covering the whole doorway. I liked the old door, also, because it was so heavy and solid; its weight made it swing slowly on its hinges, and when it shut it made a deep soft thud. That affirmative, protecting sound is one of the many things which were good and comforting in my house, and which are sweet to remember long afterward.

As soon as this treasure had been hung again on its hinges I spoke to Frank Grindle about scraping it to get off the years' accumulation of dry blistered paint which disfigured its surface. I could see in my mind's eye how wonderful the panels and the moldings would look after they had been all scraped clean, sandpapered, rubbed smooth, polished, and freshly painted—how the door would glow and shine under the fanlight, between the fluted pilasters. I waited very eagerly to see this process begin. Then I came upon Frank Grindle at work on the door, and my eagerness changed to dismay as I watched him, and saw how he dug into the wood and gouged the delicate moldings. He was working with his characteristic, rough, nervous speed, and he didn't realize what harm he was doing. He always seemed pleased when I came where he was working, and he began to beam and talk to me. But I couldn't listen because I was watching every sharp zigzag of the tool in his hand, and I winced as I saw it split off precious edges of molding and make irreparable grooves in the panels. He had been wonderful at slapping paint onto clapboards all over the outside of the house and getting it done quickly, but I saw that he was not the man for my door.

I was always extremely polite to everybody who worked for me, or at least, I believe I was, because I couldn't help being, and if any criticism was required I didn't know how to express it, because of the politeness and admiration I had established. And of course I especially liked and admired Frank Grindle so much that I couldn't bear to criticize him. So I made some kind of faltering suggestion to him about his being a little gentler with the door, but I said it so weakly and apologetically that he didn't even hear me and he raced ahead, while I suffered. I almost persuaded myself, in order to bear it, that I was mistaken, and that he was doing the scraping as any painter would do it, that the old wood was rotten and bound to give way. But I knew better and I couldn't forgive myself for my weakness in letting him go on at all, and somehow in the end I managed to find some miserable indirect way of taking him away from the door before he had quite finished the scraping job, which I then gave to Joel Perkins to do.

Lorna had told me about Joel Perkins as the man for inside painting and for papering. He was an expert, everyone said. His father had been one of the finest painters and paperers of his generation in Castine, and he had trained Joel. The Goodwins had told me he was very clever at mixing paint and could match any color perfectly. He came to see me and I found him youngish middle-aged, saturnine, and cynical looking, and very silent, with green eyes and heavy black hair which fell over his forehead.

He took charge of the door and said nothing, but his saturnine silence and his quietly observant glance at the damage done told me all I needed to know about his craftsmanship. There was something profoundly reassuring in Joel Perkins's attitude toward the door—in the intimate awareness which his hands and eyes created between himself and the thing he was working on. Watching him, I could feel an almost unlimited faith in the restoring power of a little rag of sandpaper in his fingers, rubbing back and forth over the wood. I didn't perceive in him any love of his craft or any kind of warm feeling toward it. He was too cynical for anything like that

212

—what he had was an inherited aptitude for it and a sort of cold-blooded pride in it which he had acquired from his experience and skill.

I felt very queer between these two men, Frank Grindle and Joel Perkins. Frank Grindle had a sensitive, eager, mental awareness of another person as an individual, and yet he hadn't a bit of the kind of limited, specialized, focused awareness Joel Perkins had, and consequently he had almost ruined my door without even realizing it. I was grievously torn by this situation, because I was unable to compromise with my own standard of workmanship, especially as it affected any part of my project of transformation; and yet I was unwilling to do harm to my friendship with a rare person by pointing out any fault in his work.

But I needn't have felt so troubled. Frank Grindle couldn't do any one thing long at a time. I think some dreadful nightmare was in his unconscious, always pursuing him, and he continually escaped it with his nervous speed going on to the next thing. His gay, arch face and his really sweet benign smile hid some invisible, desperate tightrope walk he was doing above an invisible abyss. So it made him too nervous to be just a painter all the time, like Joel. He was sometimes a painter, and sometimes a fisherman, always darting back and forth between two trades. As I remember, the scallop-fishing season opened the first of October, and while he was still working on my door he was in a hurry to get out into the Bay in his boat. With his usual verve and eagerness he had been telling me all about scallop fishing, how the men went out with draggers on their boats and gathered the deep-sea scallops and shipped them "to the westward"—as Castine people say when they mean Boston, New York, and Philadelphia. He described to me how the scallops are able to move and skim along very fast over the sea floor. He asked if I had ever seen a real, big, deep-sea scallop. I said I hadn't, and a few days later he brought an enormous one for me, alive, inside its classic, pilgrim's shell. This beautiful, ancient symbol, taken cold and dripping out of the waters of my own bay! Lorna opened it and cooked it for me, and I never tasted anything sweeter. The giver seemed very much pleased that I liked it so much, and I kept the two matching shells for a long time afterward.

In the meantime Joel finished the door and painted it a rich green-blue. And apparently there was no hard feeling between him and Frank Grindle. He mixed paint while I watched until he got the exact color I had in my mind's eye. After he did the door he painted all the blinds the same green-blue. So the door was finished and its beauty shone forth just as I had hoped it would, and the blinds were all dry and rehung on their hinges when the cold weather came and stopped the work. Everything we had started to do that fall was finished, and all that remained to be done before the house could be lived in was the painting of the woodwork inside the house, and the papering. And these would have to wait for the spring.

It had seemed as if that marvelous creative autumn might last forever. The sweet still air and the shrill piping of crickets and the hazy blue of the harbor seemed fixed and eternal. Then one morning we woke up to find a cold wind blowing—a wind that had an unfamiliar knife-edge in it, something we had forgotten existed. With that sudden searching cold, all the softness and the haze and the mellowness were gone. Lorna had a fire crackling in both her stoves, in kitchen and parlor. The snapping sound and fragrance of the fires on that first cold morning made the idea of winter seem very delicious, and exciting. The first wintry weather lasted several days. The men came and collected their tools out of my house and said good-by to me. I hated to have that part of my experience come to an end. This, my first independent venture into the external world of reality, had been the happiest period I had ever known.

With what must have seemed to the Castine workmen an even more amazing worldly precociousness and independence than I had yet shown, I asked them all to present their bills to me, and as soon as they did I paid them, writing out the largest cheques I had ever written in my life. And it was not only the Castine people who treated me, that autumn, like a very bright child, but my mother and Warren did the same, for I received from them surprised and gratified letters in which they commended me for what they considered my able handling of the purchase and alteration of my house. By some fortunate circumstances, neither of them was free to come and help me. And I continued my enterprise in almost complete independence.

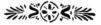

28

AFTER buying the house and paying for the repairs I planned that I would have enough money left over, if I spent it with care and forethought, to give the house a few rich touches. I was glad that the papering had to wait until spring, because I was planning to spend a luxurious length of time during the winter going to the most expensive shops in Boston where I would gaze and gaze at all sorts of beauties, and go away and come back again and meditate and not make my choice until I had looked at everything.

By using restraint in most things I intended to be joyfully unrestrained in a few. I tried to weigh and balance each improvement in its relation to the whole, in order to make each expenditure count its utmost and make my limited sum of money go as far as possible. For this was always my favorite way of doing things. I could never work with great spirit in any material unless I knew that the amount of it was limited—I had to be hedged in by a boundary of either space or material, in order to awaken the feeling of creative excitement. My favorite problem in any medium was to play freely in a strict boundary. I wanted whatever I was doing to be like a ballet, in which the boundary has to be constantly borne in the mind of the dancer, yet must appear to be forgotten in the passion and caprice of the dance. In order to fill a given limited space with his meaning the artist needs to keep himself controlled and uncontrolled all at the same time—the equilibrium between form and spontaneity must be maintained every moment or the whole thing will be ruined. To make something wonderful out of almost nothing was the favorite magic of my bedridden childhood, a magic which had been bequeathed by the child to the person I afterward became. Although I forgot it over and over, as spoiled grown-up people continually forget the gifts they possessed as unspoiled children, this one which I had enjoyed so many times was always returning to me and seeking me out, it seemed, in order to give me again its special intense satisfaction.

Now, in the enterprise of my house, I had more space and scope and liberty of action than I had ever dreamed of having before. Until now I had been in sole command of my own tools, my own small secret material, but of nothing else. Now I had a great deal, instead of nothing, to work with. Now house and land and money were mine, and I was all alone, planning and directing the work, with nobody to thwart or discourage me. It was a calm unfolding of new powers which I had never dreamed of having. It was most wonderful because it was so calm. But even now I still remembered my boundaries. I kept faithfully turning back and forth from drunken exultation in the unlimited possibilities of my new treasure to sober concentration on the limits represented in my bankbook. This duality, self-imposed, gave me a wonderful feeling of exquisite equilibrium, like walking perfectly calmly in mid-air. It was not the same magic as making something out of nothing. This was a new magic on a larger scale. But even so, one had to remember that it was magic, and that equilibrium was involved and therefore one had to step carefully.

Until I felt this unprecedented elation I had never thought of myself as having any desire to do any of these particular things. In the past I had looked with scorn at any lust for household establishments and possessions. For instance it had always been a mystery to me why people who had fallen in love should feel they must wait before they could fulfill their love till after they had gotten together an elaborate collection of household goods. I should have thought they would have preferred to pick up hastily only the bare essentials of their life together almost like the boy and the girl under the pine tree. I thought that if I were in their place I would prefer to let marriage take me at once to a room in the slums with nothing but a bed and a table and two chairs. For just as Picasso and van Gogh and others, whose painting seems even more alive than things born of the flesh, used to live and work in some barren studio where anything beyond the minimum of physical comfort and adornment seemed a nuisance and obstacle, so, I thought, that subtle love, who is also such an artist and creator and genius, needed only a very plain and simple place in which to make a beautiful and living marriage.

I had believed that the best things are made out of nothing. I was afraid that nothing might come out of too much. The motive of asceticism is to free creative energy, and its function, like that of pruning, is to make for a great flowering. The word asceticism has a harsh sound in our ears because in our time its real creative purpose has been overlooked. Our modern religion has been to possess, not to create. In contrast to this love of possessions, the bareness of my own previous life, which I had instinctively desired and which must have seemed to any observer so terribly mistaken and meager, was as I hoped the preliminary bareness of a branch that needs to be pruned so that its flower when it comes forth at last may be really something to see. For I was at that time secretly and humbly and exclusively intent on my writing. I only, no other, saw then the flower which my pruned branch bore, for I knew it wasn't good enough yet to show to anyone else. But to me, even then, it was exceedingly beautiful. It was beautiful and exceedingly wonderful, not for what it looked like in the bud, but because I alone knew the great secret about it, that it was really alive. In those years I was secretly "carrying a child," and I felt as Thomas Hardy felt in the seventies, and I had copied this poem of his in my notebook:

In the seventies I was bearing in my breast,
　　Penned tight,
Certain starry thoughts that threw a magic light . . .
　　Aye, I bore them in my breast
　　Penned tight.

In the seventies when my neighbors—even my friend
　　Saw me pass,
Heads were shaken, and I heard the word, "Alas . . ."

In the seventies those who met me did not know
　　Of the vision
That immuned me from the chillings of misprision...

In the seventies naught could darken or destroy it,
　　Locked in me,
Though as delicate as lamp-worm's lucency;
Neither mist nor murk could weaken or alloy it
In the seventies!—could not darken or destroy it,
　　Locked in me.

I couldn't have been so rapt and intent if it hadn't been for my unencumbered, empty, personal life. In contrast to my brothers and sister, who were all married then, I was deeply thankful for all I lacked. I exulted because the lack in my life of any personal meaning or possession heightened the awareness of my mind, just as the bareness of a nun's cell makes for visions. I had known such a fierce and tremendous craving for life and experience, and had received such a shock at the discovery that it was not meant for me, that I attempted to cast this reality away from me with all the passion with which I would have seized it if I could; and I balanced this violent act of rejection by flinging myself down into my writing, in recompense and adoration, in order that it might become reality's mystical counterpart.

But at last the time bomb went off which transported me to Castine, made me mistress of a house, and launched me on my great dream of what I was going to do, now that my turn had come. As I studied the figures in my bankbook of my remaining cash, and made lists of the things I was going to buy for the house, the intoxicating pleasure I felt in my possession was a new and astonishing thing.

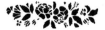

29

ALTHOUGH I was in sole command of everything concerning the purchase of the house and the changes I was making in it, I realized that in the matter of its furniture I would have to defer to my mother. We had a houseful of furniture in the Salem storage warehouse, including a number of American antiques which my mother had lovingly collected. It would clearly be a kind act to rescue all these from the tomb and bring them to a house where they could come alive again in rooms which would make them look more beautiful than ever before.

My mother consented to this plan, and a huge mover's van drove into Castine in the dead of night near the end of October, and stood at the foot of my brick path while the men unloaded the things and carried them in. I had dressed hurriedly and gone over from Lorna's, where I was sleeping. The movers were strange nocturnal beings and they insisted on unloading at once. They needed me to stay by the front door and tell them where to put each piece of furniture as it came along the path.

It was about two o'clock when they began to take the tarpaulin off their load and untie the ropes that held it. The night was mild and cloudy, with vague moonlight among the clouds. As I stood waiting, and felt the soft night wind blow against me, I looked up at the sky and all around wonderingly to find out how my domain would seem to me at that unknown hour. I felt something like Gabriel Oak in *Far from the Madding Crowd,* whose occupation of shepherd sometimes gave him a chance to study the aspect of things out of doors when all the rest of the countryside was fast asleep.

At first I found it peaceful and amusing. I could see the tall dark truck towering up into the horsechestnut tree with mysterious figures and flashlights moving over it. The scene might easily have been that of some nocturnal adventure out of Hardy, with me for the Hardyesque observer. I remembered that the emergency which usually kept Gabriel Oak awake and watchful under the night sky was the suffering of one of his ewes at lambing time. And when my quiet watchfulness was interrupted by the sudden rushing toward me of a large dark object, accompanied by the heavy breathing of the men on each side of it, and I recognized my mother's mahogany sideboard looming up in front of me, I felt as if I were acting as a sort of midwife too—like Gabriel Oak, assisting at one of Nature's strange and awful acts of disruption.

I watched them come along the path, one after another, the intimate and familiar objects which had surrounded me and all of us during our childhood and youth, and, unlike Gabriel, I felt guilty and scared. Because this, as far as I saw, was not Nature, it was only me. What had I done? Something monstrous, I thought. What a piece of egotism and effrontery, I said to myself fearfully, as I saw again after their five-year banishment from our sight my mother's dearest, most intimate possessions, my father's books, the engravings my mother and father had bought in Germany, the three Heppelwhite chairs from Baltimore that my mother had always loved so, the long, mahogany sofa, the sideboard, and all the trunks filled with more treasures. I recognized the little, old-fashioned trunk which had belonged to my mother's mother, whom we children never knew, although her grave, beautiful face was familiar to us in daguerreotypes. Her little trunk with its rounded top held, I knew, the silk dresses with great full skirts which looked so rich and heavy in the daguerreotypes and were now so tender from the passage of time that they almost turned to powder if we touched them. It held her soft linen handkerchiefs, her cream-soft underclothes and nightgowns, every piece edged with intricate hand-worked embroidery in designs of birds and flowers. I recognized too the little old-fashioned trunk with foreign labels on it that had gone to Berlin with my mother for her marriage there. Inside that one, I knew, were my mother's satin wedding shoes and her tiny, absurd wedding corset, and the heavy silk stockings with clocks on them, bought in Paris for her trousseau. I saw, as they passed by me in open baskets and boxes, our collection of children's books, our old toys and games, even the colored paper mats we wove in kindergarten, our earliest drawings. There in the middle of the night I caught a glimpse of a butterfly painted by Warren when he was four or five, an apple sewed in cardboard with red wool by Lurana—these childish things had been kept and treasured by my mother, and they now survived the present upheaval with the almost unbearable, irrelevant intimacy of personal things washed ashore after a shipwreck. When I saw all these sacred objects being so unceremoniously handed out of the mountainous truck beside the horse-chestnut tree and rushed along the brick path into a strange house in this far-off unknown place which was wholly unrelated to our past life and to the other members of the family, and all of it being done in docile obedience to my wild adventurousness, my force and desire, I was aghast at myself.

I felt stricken because of what I had done now to my mother. She had yielded to me so passively and quite blindly in this disposal of her possessions. She had never even seen this house. She had always loved and revered things, her things. She had also loved the house she bought in Danvers, the house where we all had grown up among these now familiar things. Whenever in the past I tried to explain that even though I was not married I must go away from Danvers she had always spoken of her house and her things as an obstacle to any plan I suggested. She always made some protest to my need to leave her, and presented a number of valid, realistic objections for me to dispose of first, if I could. I kept saying sulkily, people are more important than things; lives are more important than houses. I had no ability to express my point of view and make it sound right. Because I was stubborn, though so unconvincing, she tried to appease me, by reluctantly closing the house one or two winters, thinking that after a year or two I would be content to come back and live there. Appeasement failed and at last she sold the house and put her precious things in the warehouse—an event which filled every other child of the family with nostalgic sadness, although they all were married and had homes and things of their own. Only I was ruthless and unmoved by it.

Now it seemed like the meekness or the weakness of despair and exhaustion that had made her take all her things out of the warehouse again and send them to me without a word of protest, without a single objection. She had surrendered to me, I felt, as a weary parent surrenders to a hopelessly spoiled child. I felt stricken, because this yielding seemed to tell me that at last she had washed her hands of her treasures, and she had washed her hands of me—her treasure. I was, or I had been, her treasure, I knew. She had said once, "I love you better than I love my own life. If anything should happen to you I would die." When these words spurted out of her, almost against her will — difficult, painful words — I felt humble in the presence of great feeling. And I loved her fiercely too, but mine also had to be a maternal, strong, protecting love. I couldn't accept the role of the passive, clinging child. To be the object of pure classic feeling such as hers and so strong, at the time when I was longing to be free, made me embarrassed and sulky. I had edged away farther and farther, evasive and guilty. Now I was standing beside my own front door all alone. My mother had yielded to me in everything, and I felt the queer defrauded loneliness that suddenly comes upon a person who has been overindulged and is thereby set apart from ordinary people and cheated of his natural and normal place in the world. This feeling made me very much afraid for a minute, standing alone in front of my house, in the midst of my monstrous act.

Then I remembered that I couldn't let fear decide things for me, when there was no reasonable ground for being afraid. Every step I had taken during the last few years, even those which seemed most indecisive and fearful, appeared now to have been leading me to that door. Each of those previous steps had been accompanied and all but stopped by the same sense of shame and apology as I felt now, an often groundless fear of injuring someone else, or of interfering with other peoples' plans and desires. But, in opposition to the fearful misgivings, there had always been something else, quite different, working in me—the thing I first began to be conscious of when I decided to buy the house and which I then began to think of as my magic or as my little voice, and in which I believed just enough more than I believed in fear and diffidence to choose it instead of fear. Earlier in my life there had sometimes been on the side of magic only the smallest possible margin over fear, and many times it was the other way; but with almost every vital decision I had chosen magic, and every time I chose it the magic in me grew, so that the next time it was a little stronger and more willful than before.

So I told myself, standing in front of my house, it wasn't a monstrous act, it wasn't effrontery and egotism which had brought me there. I had started out long ago with a predicament to solve and in order to solve it I had gone forth on a lonely voyage of discovery—not as other people go forth openly in plain sight into the world of experience to do well or badly, but I had gone out unseen, in the little boat of my imagination, seeking in solitude and by reflection more knowledge and understanding of human experience, hoping that they might give me the wide horizon my eyes longed to behold, and that they might give me also the feeling that in my solitary boat I was voyaging through real seas, like the others. Now, in my search, magic had intervened. My little voice had guided me and in obedience to it I had come to an unknown, unexpected island. When I beheld it suddenly there in front of me, I fell in love with it, and in excitement and joyous surprise I threw away my faithful little boat and climbed ashore. I had reached at last the period of adorable, actual experience into which my quiet life was going to explode—that fascinating, little, volcanic island, almond-shaped, which lay across the fate line in the palm of my right hand.

"Sarn," Blue Hill, Maine

1935-1942

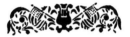

EPILOGUE: *The rest is waiting*

I FIRST began to tell my story because I needed to express my thanks for the things that have happened to me. In the beginning I said to someone, this book is going to be my bread-and-butter letter to God. I was ashamed to be saying anything about God seriously and so I had put it in a whimsical deprecating way in order to say it at all.

And because of my ignorance and stupidity, characteristic of a generation that was much too bright and clever, my voyage of discovery had to be a long and dangerous one before it began to dawn on me where my little voice came from, and what the object of my search might have been called by a better-instructed person.

Now it isn't only the others like me, still too bright to know God and too clever to kneel down, who are, unconsciously, the enemies of faith in God. There is no more time left now for us to learn slowly, because the new and conscious enemies of Christianity are doing their work so fast. But there are people willing actually to die this very afternoon because events have shown them—what they didn't know before—that they must disbelieve in man's tyranny, and that they do believe in God's guidance and in the teachings of Christ, and not in the teachings of antichrist. And there is no time left at all for anyone to learn these things slowly.

The Little Locksmith

A friend of mine in Castine named Mary Camp once remarked to me that nobody in our generation could mention God out loud except as a swearword without feeling as much embarrassment as our parents had felt at the mention of sex. That was true of me and most of my friends, and therefore I had nothing but the incorrect and evasive name of magic or my little voice when I wanted to describe the mysterious inrush of joy which at every time of decision finally came, if I waited selflessly and humbly for it, and told me which way to turn.

Now I have told part of my story, and I certainly want to tell the rest if God wills it and if enemies do not interrupt me. My upstairs workroom in a seacoast village, not very far from Castine, on the North Atlantic, is as peaceful as a monastery. While I am working I can watch the lazy woodfire burning in the fireplace and feel its sweet warmth. Every little while my husband, Dan Hathaway, cheerfully rushes in with a fresh armful of wood and puts on another log. When I get up and walk around the room in the pauses of writing I go to the low mantelpiece over the fireplace and look at the row of little shells which lie there in order, each one separate so it can be seen and admired alone. These little shells came from Mr. Moorman of Captiva Island in Florida. I sent for them one snowy February day a year and a half ago because I saw Mr. Moorman's advertisement in the *Saturday Review of Literature,* and because I love shells. I remember how exciting it was when the box came, and the fine white Florida sand began to fall out of the tissue paper as I unwrapped them. I laid them out here in a row on the dark slate-colored mantelpiece, and I love to stand and stare at them, and wonder at them for being such perfect little works of art, such enchanting shapes and decorated so stylishly, with delicate fine stripes, dots, and squares of one color upon another. I like to take one in my hand and feel it against my palm and fingers. The shells and the fluttering fire below give forth a calming pleasure in my moments of undue and sometimes painful exaltation in the midst of writing. There is a mystery, and intimacy, and a mignonne charm about the little shells which I feel whenever I go near them; it is something about them which makes them always seem alive, and refreshing to the mind.

After I have stood still and looked at my shells I walk around the room a minute, and when I look through the windows I see the harbor and our apple trees. This is the first cool day of autumn. A northwest wind is whirling around our house, shaking the trees and throwing green apples down on the grass with a thump; one of the wicker garden chairs has been blown upside down. The harbor is an intense, ruffled blue, running under this wind, and where the tide has gone out millions of wild ducks are sitting on the shiny mudflats in the sunlight. Close to my workroom window the slim, tall crab apple tree is almost blinding, it is so bright, its branches filled with ruby-red crab apples.

This is wonderful! How did I come by it? It is another house and another story. Everything is different since Castine. Yet it all began there. For there and then I first began in utter ignorance and naïveté to heed the little voice which spoke to me and told me which way to turn. This story of what happened is my song of praise and thanksgiving for the gift of life and for the little voice which kept on speaking so patiently to me, even though I was inattentive and stupid for so long. It is a song of thanksgiving, because every time I followed the lead of the little voice, even though the way it wanted me to go almost scared the life out of me, the action turned out to be a fertile action, out of which my life unfolded and grew; just as the vine on one end of our brick house, by putting out its small knowing hands, spreads little curving chains of bright-green leaves over the wall, going first one way and then another way, until it spreads knowingly its whole intricate, beautiful pattern all over the wall.

I am certainly much too ignorant still to do anything more than tell my story, and tell what I found. I knew as soon as I found it that it was the real, though unconscious, object of my search. The thing I found is a sequence. It is very simple. First, I looked, and I began to see what was in front of me. Perhaps I looked with more desperateness than a normal person does, for as Mary Webb wrote in *Precious Bane*, "When you dwell in a house you mislike, you will look out of a window a deal more than those that are content with their dwelling." At any rate, I really looked, and sometimes I think I really saw, as an artist sees, as if it were the first dawn of my life. Then, inevitably, as will happen to anyone who looks as if for the first time, I noticed that what I saw was amazing, beautiful. The beginning of the sequence, then, is, first you see, then you admire. Next admiration leads with the same inevitableness to gratitude, next, gratitude leads to humility, for the person who receives much feels grateful and then humble, because he wonders how he can have deserved such an extravagant kindness. Humility is naturally followed by a feeling of wonder and adoration toward the source of these miracles, the God who made them and put them there. Next I began to realize that marvelous things to look at are only the beginning of admiration. Not only were extraordinary treasures put before me, but, as in everyone else, in me were implemented the senses with which I am made able to respond to them and receive them. My eyes give me the delight of looking at the shapes and colors of shells; my hand, being so alive and aware, gives me the exquisite ability to put out my fingers and hold the shell and feel its shape and quality. I am even so generously supplied with senses that they complement and almost duplicate each other, so that if one is injured another can serve instead. Even if I had no hand, and no hearing, my eyes could bring me the pleasure of shells.

Besides giving me the incredibly subtle devices of the senses, the Mind of God, who imagined and made us, has added the even more intricate, mysterious, and certainly divine gift, the human mind, which widens my understanding and increases my response to the things which are in front of me away beyond the reach of the subtle senses. As if this were not enough, the mind has for companion the heart.

And although everything appears to have been planned to make us feel at home on the earth, and in possession of the earth as our own, our bodies being designed for perfect adjustment to earthly existence, if not at certain times and places for rapturous harmony with it, aren't we really in the position of guests? We came from we do not know where, and we return we do not know where.

And in that case, what incredibly rude guests!

Taking all this for granted, and then complaining, and cursing God and asking for more! Not only that, but even quick to toss it all away if there is any personal flaw or difficulty.

When I thought of our incredible rudeness I tried to think of some way to make amends and it dawned on me then to pray. That, then, is what prayer is for! I thought. It is the natural expression of those who are not so stupid and so rude as to have forgotten that they are guests. Those naïve, medieval people—and they exist always in every generation, usually obscure, unknown, and even ignorant—who begin and end each day in that most beautiful instinctive human attitude, the attitude of the sensitive, courteous guest of God, on their knees with the head bent down before an ever-present God toward whom their hearts open like drooping flowers or like radiant flowers—they are the only people who really understand admiration and gratitude. They know even more than the artists do because they know the whole of the sequence. They know the end as well as the beginning. They do not only see, and admire, and take, and stop there. In recognition of what they have seen, admired, and received, they finish the sequence, they put themselves and their lives into God's hands to do as He will with them. It seems as if perhaps these are the only people who are civilized enough, in the highest sense, to have been invited to live on the miraculous earth and to wear the miraculous human body.

It is disappointing to realize that the artists and writers, being specially endowed as they are to see and admire, are among the ones responsible for the fatal breaking of the sequence. We fell in love with ourselves and our works, and forgot our manners. We were grateful, but not grateful enough. We became more and more greedy, harder to please, we wanted everything. We never thought of kneeling down and trying to know God's will. Shockingly arrogant, ill-bred guests, we took what we wanted, if we could get it, whether it was offered to us or not, and we forgot to guard our happiness with humility and prayer. And now the entire miracle of the earth is being stolen by thieves and murderers, and a great part of the human race who possessed too much and took too much for granted is already homeless and enslaved.

If this Dark Age now covering half the earth is destined to engulf all continents and all people for centuries to come, the next new dawn that breaks upon the ruin of today's world will surely begin to shine with a tender clear light at the moment when some future wanderer lifts up his head and sees something as if for the first time, and pauses to admire, then feels in his breast a kindling fire of gratitude and wonder and then, instinctively following the sequence, falls on his knees to worship the mystery and to give himself to God.

We have lost that sequence, as all spoiled children and spoiled people lose it. Perhaps everything must be erased, and left in darkness for a long time; and perhaps out of the darkness a new and innocent people must emerge before the sequence can be found and lived again. But when the sequence is found by some forerunner of the next Golden Age, and is devoutly believed in again, and is lived again, when buildings like songs of praise rise from it as their foundation, when it is written again, and sung and embroidered and painted again, then those wise, naïve people, children of God, will have found morality again, and morality, laughed at and rejected now by the suicidally clever people, will be seen to be beautiful, miraculous, and the most precious thing in the world, without which we perish.

I love this book and I can hardly bear to leave it now, as I could hardly bear to say good-by to the workmen in Castine, and lock the doors of my house and leave it, that first fall. But I did say good-by to the men, they took their tools home, and a few days later I locked the doors and gave the keys to Lorna and Alvah, and I went away to wait for spring.

When I left it the house was in its most enticing stage, almost but not quite ready, with furniture, books, pictures, toys, games, interesting treasures of all kinds, dumped into it in magnificent confusion. I could not arrange the furniture, nor put anything away, because the painting and papering were not done. The house was like a great Christmas pie all stuffed full of nut meats, plums, raisins, citron, and lemon peel, which I had to leave for a while as if to blend and ripen. Not another thing could be done there until the winter was over. Reluctantly, too, I said good-by to my new friends, Lorna and Alvah, and as we said good-by, Lorna eagerly promised to let me know the first minute that the road into Castine from the Bucksport railroad station was passable in the spring.

I am leaving my story in the same condition as my house was when I left it then. Preliminary things are told, the rest is waiting, it is packed as full as a pie with treasures to be sorted out, examined, and put in order. But the probability of my being free to return to my story in the spring is less certain than the probability was then of my being free to return to my house. Then Alvah and Lorna and I never dreamed of anything except an unusually late snowstorm and a prolonged mud season as possible causes for my being delayed.

Some time ago, the editors at The Feminist Press sent me a photocopy of Katharine Butler Hathaway's memoir *The Little Locksmith* and asked whether I would write an afterword to the new edition they planned to publish. Because my own work deals extensively with illness, disability, and death, I get a good many requests to review and comment upon personal narratives dealing with these themes, a literary subgenre I've dubbed "the literature of personal disaster." As Thomas Couser has written in *Recovering Bodies*, "although our selves and our lives are fundamentally somatic, the body has not until recently figured prominently in life writing" (5). As though to make up for their tardy appearance, works recounting the body's vagaries and vicissitudes have crowded bookstore shelves in the past couple of decades. The range of conditions is broad: cancer (Audre Lorde, *The Cancer Journals*, Anatole Broyard, *Intoxicated by My Illness*), polio (Leonard Kriegel, *Falling Into Life*), amputation (Andre Dubus, *Meditations from a Movable Chair*), paralysis (Reynolds Price, *A Whole New Life*), mental illness (William Styron, *Darkness Visible,* Kay Redfield Jamison, *An Unquiet Mind*), to name only a handful of the most prominent.

The quality is similarly varied, and not all of those I'm asked to read repay my time. Having read *The Little Locksmith,* however, I replied at once that I'd love to write about it. This was no ordinary addition to the genre. This was a work sui generis: not merely an account, however vivid and absorbing, of a cripple's childhood and maturation but a nuanced inquiry into the social, psychosexual, and spiritual realities of disability, half a century

239

before disability studies emerged as an academic pursuit. None of the scholars engaged in this field, myself included, appeared to know of *The Little Locksmith*'s existence. Much younger then, I still believed that books were published and kept in print on the basis of their merit rather than their marketability, and I couldn't understand how this one could have been allowed to go out of print.

The Little Locksmith had been enthusiastically received when it was first published. Beginning in September 1942 the *Atlantic Monthly* serialized the work, bringing its author, in her last months, a welcome spate of admiration from friends and strangers alike; Coward-McCann published the book posthumously in 1943. Writing for the Book-of-the-Month Club, which chose it as a main selection, Christopher Morley predicted, "Kitty Butler's story . . . will outlive a good many more pressingly fashionable novels or reports of literary heroism." Similarly, in his review for the *New York Times,* Edward Wagenknecht predicted that *The Little Locksmith* "will be with us for some time." Yet by the time it was sent to me, it was long out of print. Even though I had concentrated on women's autobiography during my doctoral work, I had never come upon a single reference to it. It had, as most books are destined to do, vanished altogether.

Well, not quite. Someone at The Feminist Press knew about it. I heard nothing further from the editors, however, and after a while, I decided that the project had been abandoned. And, indeed, as I learned later, tracking down the heir who could give permission to reprint *The Little Locksmith* proved complicated enough that it very nearly had been. I held onto the photocopied pages, however, until a friend unearthed a copy for me in a used bookshop in, appropriately enough, Maine. Then the book itself—

dustjacket tattered, pages brittle and browning, redolent of overheated attics in old Maine houses—took up a spot in my permanent library. Smug as I felt with possessing my own copy, I still regretted that a new edition wasn't available for teaching and gift-giving. When, years later, I learned that the project had been revived, I felt as though a friend I had made long ago and far away was moving close enough to my home that I could throw her a big party and introduce her to everyone.

HERE SHE IS AT LAST!

Katharine Butler was born on October 2, 1890, in Baltimore, Maryland, and moved in 1895 to Salem, Massachusetts, where she spent a large part of her childhood. By accident of geography, I immediately felt connected to her. My own mother also grew up in Salem and also, after the loss of a father, was then raised in the relative backwater of Danvers. Growing up a couple of towns away, I shopped in the department store founded by Katharine Butler's grandfather, James F. Almy, and knew well all the places she and her brother Warren passed by and through on their youthful evening drives and canoeing trips: Topsfield, Boxford, North Beverly, and the Ipswich River. I think this sense of contact, however tangential, often accounts for an initial uprush of affection for a book and its author, though critics seldom concede so personal a response. This felt connection also explains why, although I shall not call this author Kitty, the name used by her intimates, I also shall not use Hathaway, following critical convention, or even the socially prescribed Mrs. or Ms. Hathaway. Rather, I shall refer to her as Katharine, the same name by which she often refers to herself in *The Little Locksmith*.

At the age of five, Katharine contracted tuberculosis of

the spine, also known as tuberculosis spondylitis or Pott's disease. Since the strain of *Mycobacterium tuberculosis* that possesses a particular affinity for bones and joints is carried by cows, she was likely infected by raw milk. Those of us born after milking herds began to be tuberculin-tested and milk to be pasteurized routinely may hardly recognize the disease, but it was once fairly common in children and, until the discovery of antibiotics, untreatable. The child was simply immobilized while the body overcame the infection, sometimes for years, in the hope of preventing the deformity kyphosis, otherwise known as curvature of the spine or, in less polite terms, hunchback. Thus, although the contraption Katharine describes sounds like an invention of medieval inquisitors, her doctor was, in fact, using the most advanced technology available to him and the results, horrifying as she found them on her first glance into the mirror, were far milder than they might have been.

Although she never grew taller than a "ten-year-old child," the (unattributed) foreword to a posthumously compiled volume of Katharine's work entitled *The Journals and Letters of The Little Locksmith* notes that "[h]er curvature was slight. Her head was handsome and low in relation to her shoulders. Her shoulders were wide, her hips narrow, and her legs and hands finely slim and beautiful, so that when she half-reclined she looked like a mermaid" (xi). A mermaid, no less, that seductive and fatal creature of seamen's fantasies! As an adolescent and young woman, however, she clearly didn't perceive herself in such a flattering light. Believing herself "deformed," "hideous," "grotesque," she assumed that romantic and sexual love were forbidden her. While in her thirties, in a piece called "Things Japanese," she reflected,

242

Afterword

> I had known for a long time that nobody could ever fall in love with me, because of my being like the little locksmith. I say I knew this, although I never had asked anybody if it were true, and nobody had ever told me that it was. Yet I believed that I ought to believe that it was true. It was their silence, not words, which made me believe that I was expected to believe this. No words ever were spoken, not a single word of enlightenment to help me solve and endure this inhuman predicament. (*Journals,* 72)

She believed, and grieved, and relinquished all hope for love.

Reading *The Little Locksmith* does little to contradict that impression, ending as it does with Katharine, the maiden aunt, still readying her house for writers, for her nieces, and for lovers presumably other than herself. Except for that one intriguing reference, in the epilogue, to "my husband, Dan Hathaway," bustling in to restoke the fire (230). What's this? Can there be more to Katharine's story? Indeed, there is. Yet since Katharine didn't live to write the companion book she had planned, and the volume collecting her letters and journals, published by Coward-McCann in 1946, is out of print, one can hardly read more. The journals and letters, however, do provide a portrait of Katharine's life up until the eve of her death, and I have drawn liberally from them not only for reflections that coincide with the writing of *The Little Locksmith* but also for Katharine's life beyond Castine—in Paris, in New York, and then in Maine again.

Once settled into the house in Castine, which she called Sellanraa after the place in Norwegian novelist Knut Hamsun's *Growth of the Soil,* she made friends with the artist Philip von Saltza, who introduced her to the

visiting Japanese artist Toshihiko. Fascinated since childhood by "all things Japanese," she fell in love with Toshihiko,
who brought her "a climax of health and freedom" and with
whom she enjoyed "a degree of intimacy which makes ordinary occidental relationship seem superficial" (*Journals,*
74). The effects of the relationship weren't entirely salu-
tary. She wrote in a letter to Toshihiko,

> My desire to write has gone out of me as completely as if
> it had been removed by an operation, through the potent
> action of love. I imagine it could not affect a man so, because
> art really belongs to a man as it doesn't belong to a woman.
> I feel now that it is a great mistake, a great sin against nature
> for my sex to seek fame or even without the desire for fame
> to give a life's devotion to any art except the art of living.
> (80)

Every woman artist has had to struggle against this patri-
archal myth, designed to assure her lover both the smallest competitive field and the most ample domestic comfort.
Art of living, indeed! Still, there's something poignant
about hearing these words in Katharine's voice. She was
not, after all, debarred from romantic love—in all its silliness as well as its splendor.

Toshihiko's departure for Paris left her bereft, pen-
ning the melancholy request: "Tell me something. Because
it doesn't matter and you're going, tell me one thing. Tell
me (as if I were dead and you were talking to someone else
with your hands on her breasts) what there was, once, about
me" (81). In words that seem peculiarly Japanese in their
balance and resignation, she assured him, in a letter written the next day, that the Thimble at Castine—the small
creamhouse that Katharine restored as a place for her

writing—awaited his return: "[Y]et the sense of waiting is so joined to the eternal waiting and eternal movement by Nature that it is all the same if the desired one returns or doesn't return. Do you understand? Yes, joy and grief *are one* and the same" (83). She must have sensed that he had gone for good.

Unbearably lonely in Castine, she moved from the high white house to a tiny apartment at 4 Patchin Place in New York City. There, she began psychoanalysis with Dr. Izette de Forest, with whom she remained in touch for the rest of her life. There also, she met and fell in love with Toshihiko's cousin Taro, himself an artist, who asked her to marry him and live in Japan. Returning to Japan to arrange the wedding, he was persuaded by his family to marry a Japanese woman instead. Although Katharine endeavored to endure this latest heartbreak with equanimity, "having lost that dream of going," she wrote in a letter to Toshihiko, "I feel lost, and almost in exile in my own country" (104–05). Perhaps for this reason, she decided to go to Paris and pursue her own interest in drawing.

Toshihiko was there, of course, "older, thin and academic-looking," though, as Katharine continued in a letter to her Radcliffe friend Catharine Huntington, he seemed to have lost much of his allure: "I couldn't even understand why I had ever loved him so much" (116). He helped her to find a furnished studio in Montparnasse and raved about her drawings. A few of these are reproduced among her letters and journals; and although they possess considerable charm, especially one of the Castine waterfront, they scarcely seem rave-worthy. Katharine's gifts seem to have been more verbal than visual. Nevertheless, she did work at her drawing, and even some painting, but, as she wrote in another letter to Catharine, only "halfheartedly," allowing herself to be "what I always was with [Toshihiko] —a listener, a consoler, simply a woman; and this mood is utterly contrary to creative mood" (149).

Having withstood the gray Paris winter and Toshihiko's often oppressive presence, she fled in the spring to the Haute Savoie to visit her friend Grace Thompson, who was being treated for tuberculosis in an Alpine sanatorium. Both the short narrative and the letters written during this interlude have a dreamy, hectic quality, as though Katharine's life had gone both out of focus and out of control. When Grace ran out of money, she left the sanatorium and moved into Katharine's hotel room. Grace was an "ex-Follies girl whose natural habitat is the speak-easy or night club"(219), and over Katharine's ladylike protestations, they took to hanging out in the hotel bistro, where they teased and flirted with the "*ouvriers*" (workers) building a new sanatorium nearby. Fleeing the tubercular "*malades*" (patients) they took a house with a couple of the "*ouvriers.*" "All the past has fallen off me, and I feel nothing but this enclosed magic place," Katharine wrote blissfully to Catherine (218). But in the fall, the ménage dissolved in a murky "tangle of deception" (225).

This chaotic period closed when, alarmed by word from Warren that their mother was ill, Katharine sailed for the United States. The following spring, at Catharine's home in Boston, she met Daniel Rugg Hathaway of Marblehead. She wrote, in a letter to Dr. de Forest, that Dan was "younger than I am, though not too much" and "sweeter to me than anybody else I have ever dreamed of" (240). This was 1932, the depths of the Depression, and with neither money nor jobs, they couldn't marry unless Katharine sold the house in Castine. As soon as she did so, they moved to Paris, where they could live more cheaply, and set up housekeeping as blissful newlyweds, "Mr. and Mrs. Muffet." Although the honeymoon inevitably ended—and although during a particularly rough patch in 1938 Katharine burst out in a letter, "I want to get a divorce from Dan" (302)—the relationship endured.

Katharine and Dan had taken with them their "beautiful cat, our Toupsie, whose dark shadow and plumy tail sweep across the floor" (242). Toupsie became the subject of a children's book, "Mr. Muffet's Cat and Her Trip to Paris," written and illustrated by Katharine, which Harper decided to publish with "childish and inexplicable enthusiasm" (265). Its acceptance, her first since she was a special student at Radcliffe, thrilled and heartened her. "I adore the feeling I have now," she wrote, "of having a profession I can really claim. I have more and more plans in my head for continuing the Muffets, for drawings, etc." (264).

These never came to fruition. Instead, a combination of homesickness and ill health sent her once again across the Atlantic. Dan remained in France for some months, but when medical opinion continued to forbid her return there, she sent for him. In Blue Hill, Maine, they bought the second house with which she fell in love during her lifetime: Sarn, an old brick place, "smaller and cozier" than the house in Castine but "unbelievably its equal in grandeur" (277). Since they hadn't enough money for the extensive renovations the Castine house had received, Dan did most of the work himself, slowly and lovingly, as well as cooking, cleaning, and nursing Katharine through increasingly frequent and lengthy bouts with chronic myocarditis, an inflammation of the heart.

Meantime, whenever she was well enough, she secluded herself in her upstairs workroom, described with her characteristic passion for the details of interior space:

247

Afterword

A square room with four windows, southwest corner. Old wallpaper, brown stripes—just brown, very odd, but quite studious-looking. A fireplace with quite nice mantel-piece, and a chest of drawers, daybed, wide oval table covered with all my pencils, erasers, pen knives, drawing pens, blotters, drawing ink, paint box, charcoal, etc., a low bench beside the couch where writing case and work in progress, as James Joyce calls it. Other side of couch is table holding victrola to call up past. There is a huge closet with shelves piled high with manuscript and notes and typewriter and typewriter paper. Also, portfolio of drawings, all of them. It really is wonderful. Windows look out into apple trees and across flowery fields to harbor. (294–95)

Here, she worked away at the project she called Obma— "the initial letters of the first line in the Song of Transformations, which is my theme song" (296)—which would become *The Little Locksmith*.

She lived to see the first but not the last of the install-ments published in the *Atlantic Monthly.* In April 1942, she explained her physical situation this way:

Years ago a famous specialist who took care of me told me I must never stop doing certain exercises which kept my abdominal muscles strong. He said I would always be all right if only I did them—because in my particular case things are so out of balance that without that reinforcement and underpinning, everything goes haywire with heart and lungs, as they begin to slump with the slumping of the underpinning. And I've neglected my exercises for about two years. (328)

She resumed these exercises, but despite her protestations
of improved health, everything continued to go "haywire." "At present," she wrote from the Blue Hill Hospital
in early December, "my only comfortable posture is on the
knees with head bent down in front of me, like a snail or
an unborn child. Only then can I breathe" (342). In this fetal
curl, she traveled by ambulance to Salem, where she died
on December 24, 1942.

"I am writing something now which I really do think is the
best I can do," Katharine wrote to her brother Warren in
1935. "It is my bread-and-butter letter to God, my thanks
for a lovely visit on the earth" (280). A couple of years later,
in a letter to Toshihiko, she commented: "A book about
myself sounds terrible, but I don't think it is terrible. I think
it is good, somewhat good; not bad, at least" (313).
Statements like these, in their measured modesty, do not
reveal whether Katharine knew, as she worked on *The Little
Locksmith,* just how remarkable the product would be. It
had, as N. E. Monroe wrote in the *Catholic World,* "unusual charm and freshness and a perceptiveness not often
found in contemporary writing." Wagenknecht explained
why he had opened his *New York Times* review with ref-
erences to Walter de la Mare, Marie Bashkirtseff, Katherine
Mansfield, William Blake, and John Keats: because *The Little
Locksmith,* "the very opposite of a derivative book[,] . . .
comes so fresh out of life, and falls so clear of established
classifications, that the only way the reviewer can give the
prospective reader a taste of its quality is thus to offer some
suggestion of the company in which it must take its place."
   The reviewer's task is to allow readers to taste a book's
quality, but space generally doesn't permit an analysis of
the complicated flavors that account for its particular

piquancy. Thus, reviewers may point out that this is an absolutely original book without revealing just how it diverges from its predecessors. As critical readers, you and I have been given more latitude for pondering what makes *The Little Locksmith* more than an ordinary memoir, and for me its distinguishing—and rather startling—characteristic is that in it Katharine has written frankly about the body. This task does not, on the face of it, seem hard to do, and plenty of books have purported to carry it out, but I would argue that precious few have actually done so. Think of D. H. Lawrence's *Lady Chatterley's Lover*, its vocabulary a veritable four-letter paean to bodily functions. But it's really a book about *ideas* about the body, quite fantastical ideas, not about the plain old carcass and its way of being in the world. Unless they dress it up in veils of metaphor and view it from some distance, most writers, like most people in general, view the body with misgiving and even distaste.

Women have long had more difficulty in writing directly about the body than have men, as Virginia Woolf points out in a classic passage from "Professions for Women": her writer's creative dream is dashed when she thinks of "something, something about the body, about the passions which was unfitting for her as a woman to know," her work brought to a standstill "by the extreme conventionality of the other sex" (61, 62). The accuracy of Woolf's critique is borne out by Monroe's report, in the *Catholic World* review, that the author of *The Little Locksmith* "has been condemned for her preoccupation with sex." Nearly sixty years later, most of us would be tempted to hoot at what even Monroe called a "rather exaggerated judgment." In *The Little Locksmith*, Katharine writes movingly but obliquely about the "great thing missing," which was "much too great and too beautiful for the body in which

Afterword

I was doomed to live" (168, 55), but her youthful beliefs about sexual love, as reflected in her musings about the tortoise laying her eggs and the young lovers in the forest glade, seem mystical and overblown rather than lewd (170–71, 173–74). In adulthood, she was quite capable of ribaldry, as the following verse, "Miss Vague and Mr. Penny," illustrates:

> V. "I want a boarder, I haven't any.
>   Someone like you going in and out
>   Would give me something to think about."
> P. "What are you, an old maid?" said he.
> V. "Oh, no, no!" She laughed roguishly.
> P. "Whereabouts do you live, is it far?"
> V. "Just up the road and there you are
>   There's a very high wall, so when you come
>   Just sing or whistle or even hum,
>   And I will hear you and know it is you
>   And then the next thing you have to do
>   Is ring the Sonnette beside the gate
>   And I'll try not to make you wait."
> P. "I know what I'll do, the best of all!"
>   Cried Mr. Penny, "I'll scale the wall."
> V. "Don't let the ivy catch your toes,
>   You've no idea how thick it grows!"
> P. "Don't you worry," he said, "my sweet,
>   Your boarder can jump without catching his feet!"
> V. "Oh!" Miss Vague gave a joyous squeal,
>   "I wonder how that will make me feel!"
>   They had a lovely time, I hear.
>   He stayed with her, off and on, for a year.
> (Journals, 266–67)

It may not be very good poetry or pornography, but its easy good humor suggests that, with experience, Katharine had grown comfortable—though hardly "preoccupied"—with sex.

This very experience and consequent comfort may have fueled her critics. For she writes about not just any body, not even just any woman's body, but a crippled woman's body; and anything "unfitting for a woman to know" is, as people with disabilities have always learned and continue to learn even in our "sexually liberated" age, doubly "unfitting" for her. Nice gimps don't do it—or even think about it. From her family's silence, Katharine learned "that I was not to have what was apparently considered the most thrilling and important experience in grown-up life. . . . The reason was so obvious that no explanation was necessary. The reason was there in the mirror for me to see . . . [and] nobody ever attempted to console me" (*Locksmith,* 167–68). Since Katharine enjoyed both love affairs and a marriage as an adult, we may assume that the true defect lay not in her physical appearance and capacity for erotic activity but in the social attitudes that, ignoring the myriad ways in which she was a normal woman to focus solely on her physical deformity, set her apart. Not merely apart but "above," as she well understood: "The locksmith is a symbol to people, they want it. . . . It is something precious to them—the virgin—the nonhuman person—the physically maimed is precious to them. Why? It seems to represent something to them purer, freer than they are—something extraordinary" (*Journals,* 348).

In the long run, the repression these attitudes caused may have done us a favor of incalculable value. For, like any good Freudian, Katharine reasons that "the natural craving to love and be loved turned itself into something else and found its miracle of satisfaction in my poetry" (*Locksmith*, 60). No one—especially not her mother—could bear the thought of a sexualized Katharine; everyone—especially her mother—admired artistic production. By sublimating her natural desires into her drawing and writing, Katharine both allayed her torment and attracted attention and affection from those who mattered most to her. Who can say whether the trade was fair? But her readers are the beneficiaries.

Even more crucially, repression of her ordinary desires transformed her into a person "susceptible to houses as some people are susceptible to other human beings" (*Journals,* 7). "Susceptible" is charged here romantically, even erotically. This is, after all, "A Person in Love with a House," as she titles one of her manuscripts published in *The Journals and Letters of The Little Locksmith*—or more accurately, as that piece makes clear, with two houses, a large clapboard one in Castine and a smaller brick one in Blue Hill, Maine. Katharine writes that the first experience "caused as much of an awakening in me as another person's first human love affair. I bought the house, and it changed the whole of my life. Marriage could not have done more" (*Journals,* 7). Indeed, in *The Little Locksmith* she speaks of the place in explicitly nuptial terms: "And so a kind of mystic marriage, an impregnation, took place between me and that piece of land and the buildings that stood on it" (133). Returning after her first winter away, as Katharine recounts in "A Person in Love with a House," she "felt the same shyness and agitation and exquisite delight that two people feel when they meet each other again for the first time after they have become lovers" (22). After selling her house in Castine, she experienced "that rigid sort of silent, speechless pain that is so well known to anybody who has ever suffered in a love affair" (39). And a few years later, finding the brick house in Blue Hill, she reflected, "It seemed more than I could possibly deserve—to find a second love after having known a first that seemed matchless" (48).

In both *The Little Locksmith* and "A Person in Love with a House," the house in Castine becomes a space of magical transformation, as well as a beloved other.

> People who came there discovered that their hair grew more curly than usual, their jokes more sparkling, their personal attraction more irresistible, their love more surprising. . . . Conversations were crazier and more inspired than in other places and sometimes lasted all night. Breakfast went on forever. (*Journals,* 32)

Less facetiously and more powerfully, she recalls an image perceived in the mirror hanging over the front-hall table.

> I did not see a woman. It looked more like a very intelligent gifted young boy. Nor did I see my deformity. It was not there; it had been canceled, wiped out, forgotten. There was an exultation in me so powerful that it canceled everything personal and limiting. What I saw in my reflection was the debonair, unsmiling look that you always see on the face of the artist when he is looking at himself and painting. . . . And behind that look something always burns and glows and triumphs; it is the artist's joy at work and in its prime. (*Journals,* 27–28)

In this house, Katharine could transcend the constraining identity of "deformed" woman and see herself as an artist.

Later, in the house in Blue Hill, the transformation completed itself with the writing of *The Little Locksmith.*

As a very young woman, she had written to Warren with
rueful humor, "I am overcome by a crazy yearning desire
for experience. I, of all people, am ill-fated by being made
with that instinct plugged into me—I who can hardly
walk up Conant Street pinned in hard by this dastardly
brace, without puffing and smothering like a porpoise"
(*Journals,* 54). Those who hang back in the face of adventure suffer deprivation, she was sure: "It is only by following
your deepest instinct that you can live a rich life and if you
let your fear of consequence prevent you from following
your deepest instinct, then your life will be safe, expedi-
ent and thin" (*Journals,* 94). Openness to and celebration
of experience remained strong: "I mean whatever happens
I like it, even if it kills me. I will probably like dying when
it comes," she wrote in her thirties; and shortly after her
marriage, "I really think I have lived about long enough,
having so many marvelous things to remember" (105,
245). Settled into her final house with a husband who had
"a remarkable talent for making fires burn, kettles boil, and
ovens bake . . . for making transplanted trees and flowers
flourish and grow and old furniture take on a luster" (51),
she wrote, again to Warren, "I have always had a terrible
craving for new experiences, but now at last my hunger and
thirst have been satisfied. I have had enough. I am perfectly
content, and now my one function is to sit in the chimney-
corner and tell about my adventures" (278).

In another sense, her beloved houses represent not
merely the magic crucible for self-transformation but the
person of Katharine herself. Tellingly, both are dilapidat-
ed enough when she buys them to require extensive repair
and maintenance, just as her own body has required work
and care. More significantly, she starts out looking for a
dwelling just like herself, "doll-like," *and does not buy one*

255

(*Locksmith*, 7). Instead, as we read in *The Little Locksmith,* she buys a house so large that it frightens her with its insistence that she grow into it, becoming the "responsive, gay, and brilliant woman" she knows herself to be, despite her visible disguise as "a little oddity, deformed and ashamed and shy" (68).

The most extraordinary quality of *The Little Locksmith,* I find, is the way in which, depending for its structure and progress on the most material elements—the body and its dwelling places—and employing very little religious rhetoric and no sanctimony, it achieves exceptional spiritual depth. Although Katharine intended it to be a book about Christianity, it hardly meets conventional expectations of such a project: that it be earnest, reverent, didactic, even dour. Instead, she could approach her professed subject with a light hand:

> I am amazed by the sayings of Christ. They seem truer than anything I have ever read. And they certainly turn the world upside down. They are rather decidedly akin to psychoanalysis as I've experienced it with Dr. de Forest.
>
> Probably I am just going crazy, like many other people who live in Maine all year round. (*Journals,* 291)

She was, however, deeply serious about her faith. Aware that "it is as embarrassing and difficult to use the word God in our generation as it was to use the word Sex in the previous one," she wrote to Dan, somewhat hesitantly, that "I have come to believe in God, the God of the New Testament, and I wish to try to live according to the teachings of the New Testament," and she begged him not to say "mocking things about the Christian religion" (316, 315–16).

In a letter to Dr. de Forest, she referred to "the abstract philosophical religious questions which are so much a part of me and my daily thoughts" (303). These, presented in raw form, might have made of *The Little Locksmith* a treatise rather than the luminous evocation of experience and feeling which it is. Revelatory rather than exegetical, Katharine's writing illuminates the text of the world with a theological grace: she wrote in a letter to Dan, "Every page, every paragraph has been written when I had a clean sense of God's guidance" (316). Throughout the book, she grasps as few writers do—but as the Jesus of the Gospels always does—the intertwining of the mundane with the holy, the body with the spirit. Even that most abstract of undertakings, writing, could be characterized in the earthiest of terms: *The Little Locksmith* emerged, she noted to her niece Libby, from "kind of a biological instinct; it is the turtle's eggs dropped slowly into the earth" (*Journals,* 341)—the same grave, slow dropping that, years before, had stirred her to sexual awareness.

The fabric of creation is, for Katharine, all of a magnificent piece, to be discerned moment by epiphanic moment, to be received in humility and awe as a gift— whether it offers pain or delight. "What good is my book if I don't know enough to be humble at all times, in all things?" she asked herself. "God is with me—controlling me, filling me just as much when I am suffering as when I am joyous" (*Journals,* 385). Few people ever achieve so spacious a vision. Fewer still can capture it in words. But we can and do respond to it. "When my book is published," Katharine speculated, "perhaps people will read it out of curiosity, many people; but I am afraid that of those who read it, not more than five or six will catch their breath and say, 'Oh, that is how I felt, too!' Or 'That is what I thought!'" (*Journals,* 373). I hope—and believe—that she had, with characteristic modesty, woefully underestimated our numbers!

Nancy Mairs
Tucson, Arizona
September 1999

Works Cited

Couser, G. Thomas. *Recovering Bodies: Illness, Disability, and Life Writing.* Madison: University of Wisconsin Press, 1997.

Hathaway, Katharine Butler. *The Journals and Letters of The Little Locksmith.* New York: Coward-McCann, Inc., 1946.

———. *The Little Locksmith.* New York: Coward-McCann, Inc., 1943.

Monroe, N. E. Review of *The Little Locksmith,* by Katharine Butler Hathaway. *Catholic World* 158 (Fall 1944): 507.

Morley, Christopher. Book-of-the-Month Club *News,* October 1943.

Wagenknecht, Edward. "A Shining Faith." Review of *The Little Locksmith,* by Katharine Butler Hathaway. *New York Times,* 24 October 1943: 4.

Woolf, Virginia. "Professions for Women." *Women and Writing,* ed. Michèle Barrett. New York: Harcourt Brace Jovanovich, 1979.

CPSIA information can be obtained
at www.ICGtesting.com
Printed in the USA
JSHW041515270222
23288JS00001B/1